Cardiomyopathies: Classification, Evaluation and Management

Cardiomyopathies: Classification, Evaluation and Management

Edited by **Bernard Tyler**

New Jersey

Published by Foster Academics,
61 Van Reypen Street,
Jersey City, NJ 07306, USA
www.fosteracademics.com

Cardiomyopathies: Classification, Evaluation and Management
Edited by Bernard Tyler

International Standard Book Number: 978-1-63242-069-5 (Hardback)

Printed in the United States of America.

Contents

Permissions

List of Contributors

Preface

Every book is initially just a concept; it takes months of research and hard work to give it the final shape in which the readers receive it. In its early stages, this book also went through rigorous reviewing. The notable contributions made by experts from across the globe were first molded into patterned chapters and then arranged in a sensibly sequential manner to bring out the best results.

Cardiomyopathies are defined as myocardial disease which leads to abnormal heart muscle. This book presents a complete, up to date examination of the current information available regarding cardiomyopathies. It presents the complete cardiovascular system as a functional unit, and the various contributors to this book analyze pathophysiological mechanisms from diverse viewpoints, by giving a classification, evaluation and management of cardiomyopathies. This book presents a broad overview of cardiomyopathies which will be of interest to researchers in this field.

It has been my immense pleasure to be a part of this project and to contribute my years of learning in such a meaningful form. I would like to take this opportunity to thank all the people who have been associated with the completion of this book at any step.

Editor

Classification, Evaluation and Management of Cardiomyopathies

Classification and Definitions of Cardiomyopathies

Bhulan Kumar Singh[1], Krishna Kolappa Pillai[1],
Kanchan Kohli[2] and Syed Ehtaishamul Haque[1]
[1]Department of Pharmacology, Faculty of Pharmacy, Hamdard University, New Delhi
[2]Department of Pharmaceutics, Faculty of Pharmacy, Hamdard University, New Delhi,
India

1. Introduction

Cardiomyopathies are an important and heterogeneous group of diseases. The awareness and knowledge of these diseases in both the public and medical communities historically has been impaired by persistent confusion surrounding definitions and nomenclature. Classification schemes, of which there have been many, (Thiene et al., 2000, 2004; Richardson et al., 1996) are potentially useful in drawing relationships and distinctions between complex disease states for the purpose of promoting greater understanding; indeed, the precise language used to describe these diseases are profoundly important.

Cardiomyopathies are diseases of the heart muscle, characterized by abnormality in chamber size and wall thickness, or functional contractile dysfunctions mainly systolic or diastolic dysfunction in the absence of coronary artery disease, hypertension, valvular disease, or congenital heart disease (Elliott et al., 2008). These diseases are classified as either primary or secondary. Primary cardiomyopathies consist of disorders solely or predominantly confined to the heart muscle, which have genetic, non-genetic, or acquired causes. Secondary cardiomyopathies are disorders that have myocardial damage as a result of systemic or multiorgan disease (Maron et al., 2006). Cardiomyopathies are classified traditionally according to morphological and functional criteria into four categories: dilated cardiomyopathy (DCM), hypertrophic cardiomyopathy (HCM), restrictive cardiomyopathy (RCM) and arrhythmogenic right ventricular cardiomyopathy/dysplasia (ARVC/D). These cardiomyopathies can be primary myocardial disorders or develop as a secondary consequence of a variety of conditions, including myocardial ischemia, inflammation, infection, increased myocardial pressure or volume load and toxic agents.

The definitions of cardiomyopathies presented here are in concert with the molecular era of cardiovascular disease and have direct clinical applications and implications for cardiac diagnosis. However, the classification of cardiomyopathies presented herein is not intended to provide precise methodologies or strategies for clinical diagnosis. Rather, the classification of cardiomyopathies represents a scientific presentation that offers new perspectives to aid in understanding this complex and heterogeneous group of diseases and basic disease mechanisms.

2. Definition

The term cardiomyopathy was used for the first time in 1957. Over the next 25 years, a number of definitions for cardiomyopathies were advanced. Indeed, in the original 1980 WHO classification, cardiomyopathies were defined only as "heart muscle diseases of unknown cause," reflecting a general lack of available information about basic disease mechanisms. In 1968, the WHO defined cardiomyopathies as "diseases of different and often unknown etiology in which the dominant feature is cardiomegaly and heart failure." The final WHO classification published in 1995 proposed "diseases of myocardium associated with cardiac dysfunction" and included for the first time ARVC/D, as well as primary RCM.

The American Heart Association (AHA) expert consensus panel proposed definition of cardiomyopathies is as follows: "Cardiomyopathies are a heterogeneous group of diseases of the myocardium associated with mechanical and/or electrical dysfunction, which usually (but not invariably) exhibit inappropriate ventricular hypertrophy or dilatation, due to a variety of etiologies that frequently are genetic. Cardiomyopathies are either confined to the heart or are part of generalized systemic disorders, and often lead to cardiovascular death or progressive heart failure–related disability." This definition of cardiomyopathies, similar to that reported by the European Society of Cardiology (ESC), under the auspices of the Working Group on Myocardial and Pericardial Diseases, excludes myocardial involvement secondary to coronary artery disease, systemic hypertension, and valvular and congenital heart disease.

3. Classifications of cardiomyopathies

Cardiac diseases can have an external cause, such as coronary artery disease, valve disease or hypertension, or may involve cardiomyopathies, in which the heart muscle itself is abnormal (i.e. an intrinsic cause of the disease is present in the heart muscle). The distinction between different classes of cardiac diseases are an important one to make, as cardiac diseases with similar phenotypes can have a diverse origin and may need different types of management. However, classification of cardiomyopathies is difficult, as the origin or pathophysiology is not always understood. Furthermore, at present there is no consensus on how to classify cardiomyopathies (e.g., based on origin, physiology or treatment) among clinicians.

In order to promote a uniform nomenclature and well-defined clinical patient groups, recent knowledge on underlying causes and pathophysiology of cardiomyopathies has been implemented in a cardiomyopathy classification system both on behalf of the American Heart Association (AHA) and of the European Society of Cardiology (ESC).

The AHA divided cardiomyopathies into 2 major groups based on predominant organ involvement. Primary cardiomyopathies (genetic, nongenetic, acquired) are those solely or predominantly confined to heart muscle and are relatively few in number (Fig. 1). Secondary cardiomyopathies show pathological myocardial involvement as part of a large number and variety of generalized systemic (multiorgan) disorders (Table 1). The frequency and degree of secondary myocardial involvement vary considerably among these diseases, some of which are exceedingly uncommon and for which the evidence of myocardial pathology may be sparse and reported in only a few patients. Because many cardiomyopathies may predominantly involve the heart but are not necessarily confined to that organ, some of the distinctions between primary and secondary cardiomyopathy are necessarily arbitrary and inevitably rely on judgment about the clinical importance and consequences of the myocardial process (Maron, 2008; Maron et al., 2006).

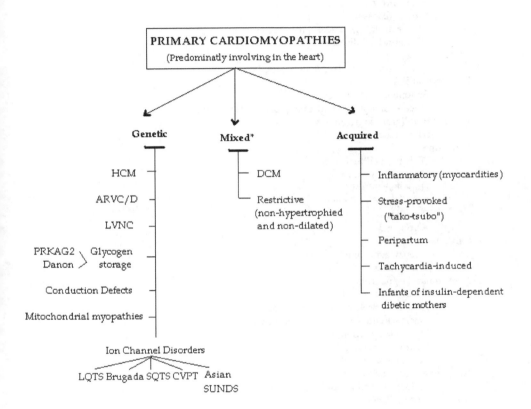

Fig. 1. Classification model for Primary cardiomyopathies (disease processes solely or predominantly involves the myocardium). The conditions have been segregated according to their genetic or nongenetic etiologies. *Predominantly nongenetic; familial disease with a genetic origin has been reported in a minority of cases. ARVC/D indicates arrhythmogenic right ventricular cardiomyopathy/dysplasia; CPVT, catecholaminergic polymorphic ventricular tachycardia; DCM, dilated cardiomyopathy; HCM, hypertrophic cardiomyopathy; LQTS, long QT syndrome; LVNC, left ventricular noncompaction; SQTS, short QT syndrome; and SUNDS, sudden unexplained nocturnal death syndrome.

Infiltrative*
      Amyloidosis (primary, familial autosomal dominant†, senile, secondary forms)
      Gaucher disease†
      Hurler's disease†
      Hunter's disease†
Storage‡
      Hemochromatosis
      Fabry's disease†
      Glycogen storage disease† (type II, Pompe)
      Niemann-Pick disease†
Toxicity
      Drugs, heavy metals, chemical agents
Endomyocardial
      Endomyocardial fibrosis
      Hypereosinophilic syndrome (Löeffler's endocarditis)
Inflammatory (granulomatous)
      Sarcoidosis
Endocrine
      Diabetes mellitus†
      Hyperthyroidism
      Hypothyroidism
      Hyperparathyroidism
      Pheochromocytoma
      Acromegaly
Cardiofacial
      Noonan syndrome†
      Lentiginosis†
Neuromuscular/neurological
      Friedreich's ataxia†
      Duchenne-Becker muscular dystrophy†
      Emery-Dreifuss muscular dystrophy†
      Myotonic dystrophy†
      Neurofibromatosis†
      Tuberous sclerosis†
Nutritional deficiencies
      Beriberi (thiamine), pallagra, scurvy, selenium, carnitine, kwashiorkor
Autoimmune/collagen
      Systemic lupus erythematosis
      Dermatomyositis
      Rheumatoid arthritis
      Scleroderma
      Polyarteritis nodosa
Electrolyte imbalance
Consequence of cancer therapy
      Anthracyclines: doxorubicin (adriamycin), daunorubicin
      Cyclophosphamide
      Radiation

*Accumulation of abnormal substances between myocytes (i.e., extracellular).
†Genetic (familial) origin.
‡Accumulation of abnormal substances within myocytes (i.e., intracellular).

Table 1. Important secondary cardiomyopathies

The ESC guidelines are more clinically orientated, which is appealing as this circumvents the complex pathophysiology of cardiomyopathies, which is not always comprehended upon presentation of the patient. According to the ESC guidelines cardiomyopathies are grouped into specific morphological and functional phenotypes; each phenotype is then sub-classified into familial and non-familial forms (Fig. 2). In this context, familial refers to the occurrence, in more than one family member, of either the same disorder or a phenotype that is (or could be) caused by the same genetic mutation and not to acquired cardiac or systemic diseases in which the clinical phenotype is influenced by genetic polymorphism. Most familial cardiomyopathies are monogenic disorders (i.e., the gene defect is sufficient by itself to cause the trait). A monogenic cardiomyopathy can be sporadic when the causative mutation is de novo, i.e. has occurred in an individual for the first time within the family (or at the germinal level in one of the parents). In this classification system, patients with identified de novo mutations are assigned to the familial category as their disorder can be subsequently transmitted to their offspring (Elliott et al., 2008). Non-familial cardiomyopathies are clinically defined by the presence of a cardiomyopathy in the index patient and the absence of disease in other family members (based on pedigree analysis and clinical evaluation). They are subdivided into idiopathic (no identifiable cause) and acquired cardiomyopathies in which ventricular dysfunction is a complication of the disorder rather than an intrinsic feature of the disease (Elliott et al., 2008).

Therefore, on the basis of all these considerations, cardiomyopathies can be most effectively classified as primary: genetic, mixed (genetic and nongenetic), acquired; and secondary.

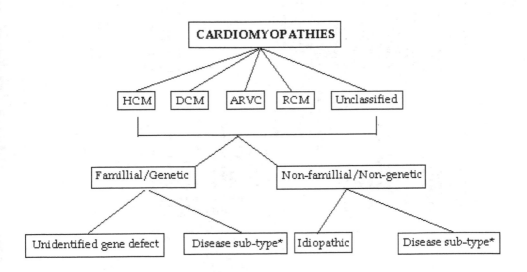

Fig. 2. Summery of proposed classification. HCM, hypertrophic cardiomyopathy; DCM, dilated cardiomyopathy; ARVC, arrhythmogenic right ventricular cardiomyopathy; RCM, restrictive cardiomyopathy (*see table 2).

	HCM	DCM	ARVC	RCM	Unclassified
Familial	Familial, unknown gene Sarcomeric protein mutations β-myosin heavy chain Cardiac myosin binding protein C Cardiac troponin I Troponin T α-tropomyosin Essential myosin light chain Regulatory myosin light chain Cardiac actin α-myosin heavy chain Titin Troponin C Muscle LIM protein Glycogen storage disease (e.g. Pompe; PRKAG2, Forbes', Danon) Lysosomal storage diseases (e.g. Anderson–Fabry, Hurler's) Disorders of fatty acid metabolism Carnitine deficiency Phosphorylase B kinase deficiency Mitochondrial cytopathies Syndromic HCM Noonan's syndrome LEOPARD syndrome Friedreich's ataxia Beckwith–Wiedemann syndrome Swyer's syndrome Other Phospholamban promoter Familial amyloid	Familial, unknown gene Sarcomeric protein mutations (see HCM) Z-band Muscle LIM protein TCAP Cytoskeletal genes Dystrophin Desmin Metavinculin Sarcoglycan complex CRYAB Epicardin Nuclear membrane Lamin A/C Emerin Mildly dilated CM Intercalated disc protein mutations (see ARVC) Mitochondrial cytopathy	Familial, unknown gene Intercalated disc protein mutations Plakoglobin Desmoplakin Plakophilin 2 Desmoglein 2 Desmocollin 2 Cardiac ryanodine receptor (RyR2) Transforming growth factor-β3 (TGFβ3)	Familial, unknown gene Sarcomeric protein mutations Troponin I (RCM +/– HCM) Essential light chain of myosin Familial amyloidosis Transthyretin (RCM + neuropathy) Apolipoprotein (RCM + nephropathy) Desminopathy Pseudoxanthoma elasticum Haemochromatosis Anderson–Fabry disease Glycogen storage disease	Left ventricular non-compaction Barth syndrome Lamin A/C ZASP α-dystrobrevin
Non-familial	Obesity Infants of diabetic mothers Athletic training Amyloid (AL/prealbumin)	Myocarditis (infective/toxic/immune) Kawasaki disease Eosinophilic (Churg Strauss syndrome) Viral persistence Drugs Pregnancy Endocrine Nutritional – thiamine, carnitine, selenium, hypophosphataemia, hypocalcaemia Alcohol Tachycardiomyopathy	Inflammation	Amyloid (AL/prealbumin) Scleroderma Endomyocardial fibrosis Hypereosinophilic syndrome Idiopathic Chromosomal cause Drugs (serotonin, methysergide, ergotamine, mercurial agents, busulfan) Carcinoid heart disease Metastatic cancers Radiation Drugs (anthracyclines)	Tako Tsubo cardiomyopathy

ARVC, arrhythmogenic right ventricular cardiomyopathy; DCM, dilated cardiomyopathy; HCM, hypertrophic cardiomyopathy; RCM, restrictive cardiomyopathy.

Table 2. Examples of different diseases that cause cardiomyopathies

3.1. Primary cardiomyopathies
3.1.1 Genetic

3.1.1.1 Hypertrophic cardiomyopathy

HCM is a condition of the heart in which a part of the myocardium or the muscle of the heart is enlarged without any obvious reasons. It is very common and affects people of all ages. HCM is a clinically heterogeneous but relatively common autosomal dominant genetic heart disease (1:500 of the general population for the disease phenotype recognized by echocardiography) that probably is the most frequently occurring cardiomyopathy (Maron, 2002). It is the most common cause of sudden cardiac death in the young (including trained athletes) and is an important substrate for heart failure disability at any age.

HCM is characterized morphologically and defined by a hypertrophied, nondilated left ventricle (LV) in the absence of another systemic or cardiac disease that is capable of producing the magnitude of wall thickening evident (e.g., systemic hypertension, aortic valve stenosis). Clinical diagnosis is customarily made with 2 dimensional echocardiography (or alternatively with cardiac magnetic resonance imaging) by detection of otherwise unexplained LV wall thickening, usually in the presence of a small LV cavity, after suspicion is raised by the clinical profile or as part of family screening (Maron et al., 2006).

When LV wall thickness is mild, differential diagnosis with physiological athlete's heart may arise. Furthermore, individuals harboring a genetic defect for HCM do not necessarily express clinical markers of their disease such as LV hypertrophy on echocardiogram, ECG abnormalities, or symptoms at all times during life, and ECG alterations can precede the appearance of hypertrophy. Indeed, virtually any LV wall thickness, even when within normal limits, is consistent with the presence of an HCM-causing mutant gene, and diagnosis can be made by laboratory DNA analysis. Furthermore, recognition of LV hypertrophy may be age related with its initial appearance delayed well into adulthood (adult morphological conversion). Most HCM patients have the propensity to develop dynamic obstruction to LV outflow under resting or physiologically provocable conditions, produced by systolic anterior motion of the mitral valve with ventricular septal contact (Maron et al., 2006).

HCM is caused by a variety of mutations encoding contractile proteins of the cardiac sarcomere. Currently, 11 mutant genes are associated with HCM, most commonly β-myosin heavy chain (the first identified) and myosin binding protein C (Barry et al., 2008; Lowey, 2002). The other 9 genes appear to account for far fewer cases of HCM and include troponin T and I, regulatory and essential myosin light chains, titin, α-tropomyosin, α-actin, α-myosin heavy chain, and muscle LIM protein (Barry et al., 2008; Selvetella & Lembo, 2005). This genetic diversity is compounded by considerable intragenic heterogeneity, with >400 individual mutations now identified. These most commonly are missense mutations but include insertions, deletions, and splice (split-site) mutations encoding truncated sarcomeric proteins (Maron et al., 2006). The characteristic diversity of the HCM phenotype is attributable to the disease causing mutations and probably to the influence of modifier genes and environmental factors.

In addition, nonsarcomeric protein mutations in 2 genes involved in cardiac metabolism have recently been reported to be responsible for primary cardiac glycogen storage diseases in older children and adults with a clinical presentation mimicking (or indistinguishable from) that of sarcomeric HCM. One of these conditions involves the gene encoding the γ-2-regulatory subunit of the AMP-activated protein kinase (PRKAG2), associated with variable degrees of LV hypertrophy and ventricular pre-excitation. The other involves the gene encoding lysosome-associated membrane protein-2 (LAMP-2), resulting in Danon-type storage disease (Maron et al., 2006). Clinical manifestations are limited largely to the heart, usually with massive degrees of LV hypertrophy and ventricular pre-excitation. These disorders are now part of a subgroup of previously described infiltrative forms of LV hypertrophy such as Pompe disease, a glycogen storage disease caused by α-1,4 glycosidase (acid maltase deficiency) in infants, and Fabry's disease, an X-linked recessive disorder of glycosphingolipid metabolism caused by a deficiency of the lysosomal enzyme α-galactosidase A, resulting in intracellular accumulation of glycosphingolipids. Undoubtedly, many other mutations causing cardiac hypertrophy by disrupting sarcomere, metabolic, and other genes remain to be identified (Elliott et al., 2008).

A number of other diseases associated with LV hypertrophy involve prominent thickening of the LV wall, occurring mostly in infants and children ≤4 years of age, which may resemble or mimic typical HCM caused by sarcomere protein mutations. These cardiomyopathies include secondary forms such as Noonan syndrome, an autosomal dominant cardiofacial condition associated with a variety of cardiac defects (most commonly, dysplastic pulmonary valve stenosis and atrial septal defect) resulting from mutations in PTPN11, a gene encoding the nonreceptor protein tyrosine phosphatase SHP-2 genes. At present, the causes of most cases of pediatric cardiomyopathies are unknown (Maron et al., 2006).

Other diseases in this category are mitochondrial myopathies resulting from mutations encoding mitochondrial DNA (including Kearns-Sayre syndrome) or mitochondrial proteins associated with ATP electron transport chain enzyme defects that alter mitochondrial morphology. Also included in these considerations are metabolic myopathies representing ATP production and utilization defects involving abnormalities of fatty acid oxidation (acyl CoA dehydrogenase deficiencies) and carnitine deficiency, as well as infiltrative myopathies, i.e., glycogen storage diseases (type II; autosomal recessive Pompe disease), Hunter's and Hurler's diseases, and the transient and nonfamilial cardiomyopathy as part of generalized organomegaly, recognized in infants of insulin-dependent diabetic mothers. In older patients, a number of systemic diseases have been associated with hypertrophic forms of cardiomyopathy; these include Friedreich's ataxia, pheochromocytoma, neurofibromatosis, lentiginosis, and tuberous sclerosis.

3.1.1.2 Arrhythmogenic right ventricular cardiomyopathy/dysplasia

ARVC/D is predominantly a genetically determined heart muscle disorder that is characterized pathologically by fibrofatty replacement of the right ventricular (RV) myocardium (Basso et al., 2009). In the early stage of the disease, structural changes may be absent or subtle and confined to a localized region of the RV, typically the inflow tract, outflow tract, or apex of the RV, the "triangle of dysplasia." Progression to more diffuse RV disease and left ventricular (LV) involvement, typically affecting the posterior lateral wall, is common (Marcus et al., 2010).

ARVC/D is a familial disease in at least 50% of cases and is typically transmitted as an autosomal dominant trait with variable penetrance. On the basis of clinical studies and data obtained from pre-participation screening for sport activity, the estimated prevalence of the disease in the general population ranges from 1 in 1000 to 1 in 5000 (Nava et al., 2000).

ARVC/D has a broad clinical spectrum, usually presenting clinically with ventricular tachyarrhythmias (e.g., monomorphic ventricular tachycardia). Noninvasive clinical diagnosis may be confounding, without an easily obtained single test or finding that is definitively diagnostic, and generally requires an integrated assessment of electrical, functional, and anatomic abnormalities. Diagnosis often requires a high index of suspicion, frequently triggered by presentation with arrhythmias, syncope, or cardiac arrest, as well as global or segmental chamber dilatation or wall motion abnormalities (Marcus et al., 2010).

Noninvasive tests used to diagnose ARVC/D, in addition to personal and family history, include 12-lead ECG, echocardiography, right ventricular angiography, cardiac magnetic resonance imaging, and computerized tomography. Endomyocardial biopsy from the right ventricular free wall is a sensitive diagnostic marker when fibrofatty infiltration is associated with surviving strands of myocytes. ECGs most commonly show abnormal repolarization with T-wave inversion in leads V_1 through V_3 and small-amplitude potentials at the end of the QRS complex (epsilon wave); Brugada syndrome–like right bundle-branch block and right precordial ST-segment elevation accompanied by polymorphic ventricular tachycardia also have been reported in a small subpopulation of ARVC/D patients (Basso et al., 2009; Protonotarios et al., 2011).

ARVC/D shows autosomal dominant inheritance, albeit often with incomplete penetrance. Autosomal dominant ARVC/D has been mapped to 8 chromosomal loci, with mutations identified thus far in 4 genes: the cardiac ryanodine receptor RyR2, which is also responsible for familial catecholaminergic polymorphic ventricular tachycardia (CPVT); desmoplakin; plakophillin-2; and mutations altering regulatory sequences of the transforming growth factor-β gene, which has a role in inflammation. Two recessive forms have been described in conjunction with palmoplantar keratoderma and woolly hair (Naxos disease) and with Carvajal syndrome, caused by mutations in junctional plakoglobin and desmoplakin, respectively. Although the function of desmosomal proteins to anchor intermediate filaments to desmosomes implicates ARVC/D as a primary structural abnormality, there is also a link to ion channel dysfunction (Maron et al., 2006).

3.1.1.3 Left ventricular noncompaction

Noncompaction of ventricular myocardium is a recently recognized congenital cardiomyopathy characterized by a distinctive ("spongy") morphological appearance of the LV myocardium. Noncompaction involves predominantly the distal (apical) portion of the LV chamber with deep intertrabecular recesses (sinusoids) in communication with the ventricular cavity, resulting from an arrest in the normal embryogenesis (Freedom et al., 2005). LV noncompaction (LVNC) may be an isolated finding or may be associated with other congenital heart anomalies such as complex cyanotic congenital heart disease.

Diagnosis is made with 2-dimensional echocardiography, cardiac magnetic resonance imaging, or LV angiography (Chin et al., 1990). The natural history of LVNC is largely unresolved but includes LV systolic dysfunction and heart failure (and some cases of heart transplantation), thromboemboli, arrhythmias, sudden death, and diverse forms of remodeling. Both familial and nonfamilial cases have been described. In the isolated form of LVNC, ZASP (Z-line) and mitochondrial mutations, and X-linked inheritance resulting from mutations in the G4.5 gene encoding tafazzin (including association with Barth syndrome in neonates) have been reported. Noncompaction associated with congenital heart disease has been shown to result from mutations in the α-dystrobrevin gene and transcription factor NKX2.5 (Monserrat Iglesias, 2008).

3.1.1.4 Conduction system disease

Lenegre disease, also called as progressive cardiac conduction defect. It is characterized by primary progressive development of cardiac conduction defects in the His-Purkinje system, leading to widening of the QRS complex, long pauses, and bradycardia that may trigger syncope. Phenotypically sick sinus syndrome is similar to progressive cardiac conduction defect. Familial occurrence of both syndromes has been reported with an autosomal dominant pattern of inheritance. An ion channelopathy, in the form of SCN5A mutations, is thought to contribute to these conduction system defects. Wolff-Parkinson-White syndrome is familial in some cases, but information about the genetic causes is unavailable.

3.1.1.5 Ion channelopathies

There is a growing list of uncommon inherited and congenital arrhythmia disorders caused by mutations in genes encoding defective ionic channel proteins, governing cell membrane transit of sodium and potassium ions (Aleong et al., 2007). These ion channel disorders include LQTS, short-QT syndrome (SQTS), Brugada syndrome, and CPVT. Nocturnal sudden unexplained death syndrome in young Southeast Asian males and Brugada syndrome are based on similar clinical and genetic profiles. A small proportion (5% to 10%) of sudden infant deaths also may be linked to ion channelopathies, including LQTS, SQTS, and Brugada syndrome (Modell & Lehmann, 2006). Clinical diagnosis of the ion channelopathies often can be made by identification of the disease phenotype on standard 12-lead ECG. Some of these cases had previously been classified as idiopathic ventricular fibrillation, a description that persists for a syndrome in which mechanistic understanding is lacking (Aleong et al., 2007; Kass, 2005).

3.1.1.5.1 Long-QT syndrome

This is the most common condition of the ion channelopathies. It is characterized by prolongation of ventricular repolarization and QT interval (corrected for heart rate) on the standard 12-lead ECG, a specific form of polymorphic ventricular tachycardia (torsade des pointes), and a risk for syncope and sudden cardiac death. Phenotypic expression (on the ECG) varies considerably, and ~25% to 50% of affected family members may show borderline or even normal QT intervals.

Two patterns of inheritance have been described in LQTS: a rare autosomal recessive disease associated with deafness (Jervell and Lange-Nielsen syndrome), which is caused by 2 genes that encode for the slowly activating delayed rectifier potassium channel (KCNQ1 and KCNE1 (minK)), and the much more common autosomal dominant disease unassociated with deafness (Romano-Ward syndrome), which is caused by mutations in 8 different genes. These include KCNQ1 (KvLQT1, LQT1), KCNH2 (HERG, LQT2), SCN5A (Na1.5, LQT3), ANKB (LQT4), KCNE1 (minK, LQT5), KCNE2 (MiRP1, LQT6), KCNJ2 (Kir2.1, LQT7, Andersen's syndrome), and CACNA1C (Ca1.2, LQT8, Timothy syndrome). Of the 8 genes, 6 encode for cardiac potassium channels, 1 for the sodium channel (SCN5A, LQT3), and 1 for the protein ankyrin, which is involved in anchoring ion channels to the cellular membrane (ANKB) (Maron et al., 2006).

3.1.1.5.2 Brugada syndrome

This syndrome is a relatively new clinical entity associated with sudden cardiac death in young people. First described in 1992, the syndrome is identified by a distinctive ECG pattern consisting of right bundle-branch block and coved ST-segment elevation in the anterior pre-cordial leads (V_1 through V_3). The characteristic ECG pattern is often concealed and may be unmasked with the administration of sodium channel blockers, including ajmaline, flecainide, procainamide, and pilsicainide. Familial autosomal dominant and sporadic forms have been linked to mutations in an α-subunit of the cardiac sodium channel gene SCN5A (the same gene responsible for LQT3) in 20% of patients. Another locus has been reported on the short arm of chromosome 3, but no gene has been identified. Sudden unexplained nocturnal death syndrome, found predominantly in young Southeast Asian males (i.e., those from Thailand, Japan, the Philippines, and Cambodia), is a disorder causing sudden death during sleep as a result of ventricular tachycardia/fibrillation. Some cases of sudden unexplained nocturnal death syndrome resulting from SCN5A gene mutations and Brugada syndrome have been shown to be phenotypically, genetically, and functionally the same disorder (Antzelevitch et al., 2005; Krittayaphong et al., 2003).

3.1.1.5.3 Catecholaminergic polymorphic ventricular tachycardia

CPVT is characterized by syncope, sudden death, polymorphic ventricular tachycardia triggered by vigorous physical exertion or acute emotion (usually in children and adolescents), a normal resting ECG, and the absence of structural cardiac disease. Family history of 1 or multiple sudden cardiac deaths are evident in 30% of cases. The resting ECG is unremarkable, except for sinus bradycardia and prominent U waves in some patients. The most typical arrhythmia of CPVT is bidirectional ventricular tachycardia presenting with an alternating QRS axis. The autosomal dominant form of the disease has been linked to the RyR2 gene encoding for the cardiac ryanodine receptor, a large protein that forms the Ca^{2+} release channel in the sarcoplasmic reticulum that is essential for regulation of excitation-contraction coupling and $[Ca^{2+}]i$ levels. An autosomal recessive form has been linked to CASQ2, a gene that encodes for calsequestrin, a protein that serves as a major Ca^{2+}-binding protein in the terminal cisternae of the sarcoplasmic reticulum. Calsequestrin is bound to the ryanodine receptor and participates in the control of excitation-contraction coupling (Wilde et al., 2008).

3.1.1.5.4 Short-QT syndrome

First described in 2000, the SQTS is characterized by a short QT interval (<330 ms) on an ECG and a high incidence of sudden cardiac death resulting from ventricular tachycardia/fibrillation. Another distinctive ECG feature of SQTS is the appearance of tall peaked T waves similar to those encountered with hyperkalemia. The syndrome has been linked to gain-of-function mutations in KCNH2 (HERG, SQT1), KCNQ1 (KvLQT1, SQT2), and KCNJ2 (Kir2.1, SQT3), causing an increase in the intensity of I_{kr}, I_{ks} and I_{kl}, respectively (Gaita et al., 2003; Schimpf et al., 2005).

3.1.1.5.5 Idiopathic ventricular fibrillation

A subgroup of patients with sudden death appears in the literature with the designation of idiopathic ventricular fibrillation. However, it is likely that idiopathic ventricular fibrillation is not an independent disease entity but rather a conglomeration of conditions with normal gross and microscopic findings in which arrhythmic risk undoubtedly derives from molecular abnormalities, most likely ion channel mutations. At present, insufficient data are available to permit the classification of idiopathic ventricular fibrillation as a distinct cardiomyopathy (Chen et al., 1998).

3.1.2 Mixed (genetic and nongenetic)

3.1.2.1 Dilated cardiomyopathy

DCM is the most common cardiomyopathy worldwide and has many causes. It is a heart muscle disorder defined by the presence of a dilated and poorly functioning left or both ventricles. It can be primary (genetic, mixed or predominantly familial non-genetic, or acquired) or secondary (e.g., infiltrative or autoimmune). This disease can be diagnosed in association with recognized cardiovascular disease; however, to qualify as DCM, the extent of myocardial dysfunction cannot be explained exclusively by abnormal loading conditions (hypertension, valve disease) or ischaemic heart disease (Elliott et al., 2008; Jefferies & Towbin, 2010). A large number of cardiac and systemic diseases can cause systolic impairment and left ventricular dilatation, but in the majority of patients no identifiable cause is found hence the term "idiopathic" dilated cardiomyopathy (IDC). There are experimental and clinical data in animals and humans suggesting that genetic, viral, and immune factors contribute to the pathophysiology of IDC (Elliott, 2000). DCM is associated with sudden cardiac death and heart failure, resulting in a large cost burden because of the very high rate of hospital admission and the potential need for heart transplantation.

DCM is characterized mainly by left ventricular systolic (or diastolic in some case) dysfunction (abnormality of contraction), with an associated increase in mass and volume. Right ventricular dilation and dysfunction can also develop but are not needed for diagnosis. Prevalence in the general population remains undefined. This disorder develops at any age, in either sex, and in people of any ethnic origin (Rosamond et al., 2008; Towbin et al., 2006). In adults, DCM arises more commonly in men than in women. In children, the yearly incidence is 0.57 cases per 100000 per year overall, but is higher in boys than in girls (0.66 vs. 0.47 cases per 100000, P<0.006), in black people than in white people (0.98 vs. 0.46 cases per 100000, P<0.001), and in babies younger than 1 year than in children (4.40 vs. 0.34 cases per 100000, P<0.001). Two thirds of children are thought to have idiopathic disease (Towbin et al., 2006). In adults, the prevalence is 1 in 2500 individuals, with an incidence of 7 per 100000 per year (but it could be underdiagnosed). In many cases, the disease is inherited, and is called familial dilated cardiomyopathy (FDC). The familial type might account for 20-48% of all cases (Taylor et al., 2006). To achieve improved care and outcomes in children and adults, a broadened understanding of the causes of these disorders are needed.

In this disease, the left ventricle is dilated, and more spherical than usual with raised wall stress and depressed systolic function. Mitral regurgitation, thromboembolic events and ventricular arrhythmias can also develop. Occasionally, other rhythm disturbances such as atrioventricular block, supraventricular tachycardia with or without pre-excitation including Wolf-Parkinson-White syndrome and atrial fibrillation develop. In the most severe cases, affected individuals present with signs and symptoms of HF–diaphoresis, breathlessness at rest or with exertion, orthopnoea, exercise intolerance, early onset fatigue, abdominal pain, and pallor. Cachexia and peripheral oedema typically arise late in the course of the disease. Young children often have poor appetite and cachexia, similar to adults. Sinus tachycardia, gallop rhythm, jugular-venous distention, pallor, cool hands and feet, hepatomegaly, and a murmur that is consistent with mitral regurgitation are common findings at physical examination (Jefferies & Towbin, 2010; Luk et al., 2009). Additionally, peripheral oedema and ascites are late signs in children. DCM can occur in a number of X-linked diseases such as Becker's and Duchenne's muscular dystrophies. It may also occur in patients with mitochondrial DNA mutations and inherited metabolic disorders. Thus when taking a family history, specific attention should be given to a history of muscular dystrophy, features of mitochondrial disease (for example, familial diabetes, deafness, epilepsy, maternal inheritance), and signs and symptoms of other inherited metabolic diseases (Elliott, 2000)

About 20-48% of DCM have been reported as familial, although with incomplete and age-dependent penetrance, and linked to a diverse group of >20 loci and genes ((Taylor et al., 2006)). Although genetically heterogeneous, the predominant mode of inheritance for DCM is autosomal dominant, with X-linked autosomal recessive and mitochondrial inheritance less frequent. Several of the mutant genes linked to autosomal dominant DCM encode the same contractile sarcomeric proteins that are responsible for HCM, including α-cardiac actin; α-tropomyosin; cardiac troponin T, I, and C; β- and α-myosin heavy chain; and myosin binding protein C. Z-disc protein-encoding genes, including muscle LIM protein, α-actinin-2, ZASP, and titin, also have been identified.

DCM is also caused by a number of mutations in other genes encoding cytoskeletal/sarcolemmal, nuclear envelope, sarcomere, and transcriptional coactivator proteins. The most common of these probably is the lamin A/C gene, also associated with conduction system disease, which encodes a nuclear envelope intermediate filament protein. Mutations in this gene also cause Emery-Dreifuss muscular dystrophy. The X-linked gene responsible for Emery-Dreifuss muscular dystrophy, emerin (another nuclear lamin protein), also causes similar clinical features. Other DCM genes of this type include desmin, caveolin, and β- and α-sarcoglycan, as well as the mitochondrial respiratory chain gene. X-linked DCM is caused by the Duchenne muscular dystrophy (dystrophin) gene, whereas G4.5 (tafazzin), a mitochondrial protein of unknown function, causes Barth syndrome, which is an X-linked cardioskeletal myopathy in infants (Maron et al., 2006).

3.1.2.2 Restrictive cardiomyopathy

RCM is defined as heart-muscle disease that results in impaired ventricular filling, with normal or decreased diastolic volume of either or both ventricles. Systolic function usually remains normal, at least early in the disease, and wall thickness may be normal or increased, depending on the underlying cause (Kushwaha et al., 1997).

The exact prevalence of RCM is unknown but it is probably the least common type of cardiomyopathy. RCM may be idiopathic, familial, or result from various systemic disorders, in particular, amyloidosis, sarcoidosis, carcinoid heart disease, scleroderma and anthracycline toxicity. Familial RCM is often characterized by autosomal dominant inheritance, which in some families is caused by mutations in the troponin I gene; in others, familial RCM is associated with conduction defects, caused by mutations in the desmin gene (usually associated with skeletal myopathy) (Fitzpatrick et al., 1990). Rarely, familial disease can be associated with autosomal recessive inheritance (such as haemochromatosis caused by mutations in the HFE gene, or glycogen storage disease), or with X-linked inheritance (such as Anderson–Fabry disease) (Elliott et al., 2008).

RCM can also be caused by endocardial pathology (fibrosis, fibroelastosis, and thrombosis) that impairs diastolic function. These disorders can be sub-classified according to the presence of eosinophilia into endomyocardial diseases with hypereosinophilia (e.g., hypereosinophilic syndromes (HES)) and endomyocardial disease without hypereosinophilia (e.g., endomyocardial fibrosis (EMF)) (Fauci et al., 1982). Parasitic infections, drugs such as methysergide, and inflammatory and nutritional factors have been implicated in acquired forms of EMF. Fibrous endocardial lesions of the right and/or left ventricular inflow tract cause incompetence of the atrioventricular valves (Kushwaha et al., 1997). Isolated left ventricular involvement results in pulmonary congestion and predominant right ventricular involvement leads to right heart failure.

3.1.3 Acquired

3.1.3.1 Myocarditis (inflammatory cardiomyopathy)

Myocarditis is an acute or a chronic inflammatory process affecting the myocardium produced by a wide variety of toxins and drugs (e.g., cocaine, interleukin 2) or infectious agents, most commonly including viral (e.g., coxsackievirus, adenovirus, parvovirus, HIV), bacterial (e.g., diphtheria, meningococcus, psittacosis, streptococcus), rickettsial (e.g., typhus, Rocky Mountain spotted fever), fungal (e.g., aspergillosis, candidiasis), and parasitic (Chagas disease, toxoplasmosis), as well as Whipple disease (intestinal lipodystrophy), giant cell myocarditis, and hypersensitivity reactions to drugs such as antibiotics, sulfonamides, anticonvulsants, and anti-inflammatories. Endocardial fibroelastosis is a DCM in infants and children that is a consequence of viral myocarditis in utero (mumps) (Maron et al., 2006).

Myocarditis typically evolves through active, healing, and healed stages. It is characterized progressively by inflammatory cell infiltrates leading to interstitial edema and focal myocyte necrosis and ultimately replacement fibrosis (Calabrese & Thiene, 2003). These pathological processes create an electrically unstable substrate predisposing to the development of ventricular tachyarrhythmias. In some instances, an episode of viral myocarditis (frequently subclinical) can trigger an autoimmune reaction that causes immunologic damage to the myocardium or cytoskeletal disruption, culminating in DCM with LV dysfunction. Evidence for the evolution of myocarditis to DCM comes from several sources, including animal models, the finding of inflammatory infiltrates and persistence of viral RNA in endomyocardial biopsies from patients with DCM, and the natural history of patients with selected conditions such as Chagas disease. The list of agents responsible for inflammatory myocarditis overlaps with that of the infectious origin of DCM, thereby underscoring the potential interrelationship between the 2 conditions (Cooper, 2009).

Myocarditis can be diagnosed by established histopathological, histochemical, or molecular criteria, but it is challenging to identify clinically. Suspicion may be raised by chest pain, exertional dyspnea, fatigue, syncope, palpitations, ventricular tachyarrhythmias, and conduction abnormalities or by acute congestive heart failure or cardiogenic shock associated with LV dilatation and/or segmental wall motion abnormalities and ST-T changes on ECG. When myocarditis is suspected from the clinical profile, an endomyocardial biopsy may resolve an otherwise ambiguous situation by virtue of diagnostic inflammatory (leukocyte) infiltrate and necrosis (i.e., the Dallas criteria) but also is limited by insensitivity and false-negative histological results. The diagnostic yield of myocardial biopsies can be enhanced substantially by molecular analysis with DNA-RNA extraction and polymerase chain reaction amplification of the viral genome. In addition to the inflammatory process, viral genome encoded proteases appear to disrupt the cytoskeletal sarcomeric linkages of cardiomyocytes (Calabrese & Thiene, 2003; Parrillo, 2001).

3.1.3.2 Stress ("Tako-Tsubo") cardiomyopathy

Stress cardiomyopathy, first reported in Japan as "takotsubo," is a recently described clinical entity characterized by acute but rapidly reversible LV systolic dysfunction in the absence of atherosclerotic coronary artery disease, triggered by profound psychological stress (Sealove et al., 2008; Sharkey et al., 2005). This distinctive form of ventricular stunning typically affects older women and preferentially involves the distal portion of the LV chamber ("apical ballooning"), with the basal LV hypercontractile. Although presentation often mimics ST-segment–elevation myocardial infarction, outcome is favorable with appropriate medical therapy.

3.2 Secondary cardiomyopathies

The most important secondary cardiomyopathies are provided in the Table 1. This list, however, is not intended to represent an exhaustive and complete tabulation of the vast number of systemic conditions reported to involve the myocardium. Rather, it is limited to the most common of these diseases most consistently associated with a cardiomyopathy.

4. References

Aleong, R.G., Milan, D.J. & Ellinor, P.T. (2007). The diagnosis and treatment of cardiac ion channelopathies: congenital long QT syndrome and Brugada syndrome. *Current Treateatment Options in Cardiovascular Medicine*, Vol. 9, No. 5, (October 2007), pp. 364-371, ISSN 1092-8464

Antzelevitch, C., Brugada, P., Borggrefe, M., Brugada, J., Brugada, R., Corrado, D., Gussak, I., LeMarec, H., Nademanee, K., Perez Riera, A.R., Shimizu, W., Schulze-Bahr, E., Tan, H. & Wilde, A. (2005). Brugada syndrome: report of the second consensus conference: endorsed by the Heart Rhythm Society and the European Heart Rhythm Association. *Circulation*, Vol. 111, No. 5, (January 17, 2005), pp. 659-670, ISSN 0009-7322

Barry, S.P., Davidson, S.M. & Townsend, P.A. (2008). Molecular regulation of cardiac hypertrophy. *The International Journal of Biochemistry and Cell Biology*, Vol. 40, No. 10, (February 26, 2008), pp. 2023-2039, ISSN 1357-2725

Basso, C., Corrado, D., Marcus, F.I., Nava, A. & Thiene G. (2009). Arrhythmogenic right ventricular cardiomyopathy. *Lancet*, Vol. 373, No. 9671, (April 11, 2009), pp. 1289-1300 ISSN 0140-6736

Calabrese, F. & Thiene, G. (2003). Myocarditis and inflammatory cardiomyopathy: microbiological and molecular biological aspects. *Cardiovascular Research.*, Vol. 60, No. 1, (October 2003), pp. 11-25, ISSN 0008-6363

Chen, Q., Kirsch, G.E., Zhang, D., Brugada, R., Brugada, J., Brugada, P., Potenza, D., Moya, A., Borggrefe, M., Breithardt, G., Ortiz-Lopez, R., Wang, Z., Antzelevitch, C.,

O'Brien, R.E., Schulze-Bahr, E., Keating, M.T., Towbin, J.A. & Wang, Q. (1998). Genetic basis and molecular mechanism for idiopathic ventricular fibrillation. *Nature*, Vol. 392, No. 6673, (March 19, 1998), pp. 293-296, ISSN 0028-0836

Chin, T.K., Perloff, J.K., Williams, R.G., Jue, K. & Mohrmann, R. (1990). Isolated noncompaction of left ventricular myocardium. A study of eight cases. *Circulation*, Vol. 82, No. 2, (August 1990), pp. 507-513, ISSN 0009-7322

Cooper, L.T. Jr. (2009). Myocarditis. *The New England Journal of Medicine*, Vol. 360, No. 15, (April 9, 2009), pp. 1526-1538, ISSN 0028-4793

Elliott, P. (2000). Cardiomyopathy. Diagnosis and management of dilated cardiomyopathy. *Heart*, Vol. 84, No. 1, (July 2000), pp. 106-112, ISSN 1355-6037

Elliott, P., Andersson, B., Arbustini, E., Bilinska, Z., Cecchi, F., Charron, P., Dubourg, O., Kühl, U., Maisch, B., McKenna, W.J., Monserrat, L., Pankuweit, S., Rapezzi, C., Seferovic, P., Tavazzi, L. & Keren, A. (2008). Classification of the cardiomyopathies: a position statement from the European Society Of Cardiology Working Group on Myocardial and Pericardial Diseases. *European Heart Journal*, Vol. 29, No. 2, (January 2008), pp. 270-276, ISSN 0195-668x

Fauci, A.S., Harley, J.B., Roberts, W.C., Ferrans, V.J., Gralnick, H.R. & Bjornson, B.H. (1982). The idiopathic hypereosinophilic syndrome: clinical, pathophysiologic, and therapeutic considerations. *Annals of Internal Medicine*, Vol. 97, No. 1, (July 1982), pp. 78-92, ISSN 0003-4819

Fitzpatrick, A.P., Shapiro, L.M., Rickards, A.F. & Poole-Wilson, P.A. (1990). Familial restrictive cardiomyopathy with atrioventricular block and skeletal myopathy. *British Heart Journal*, Vol. 63, No. 2, (February 1990), pp. 114-118, ISSN 0007-0769

Freedom, R.M., Yoo, S.J., Perrin, D., Taylor, G., Petersen, S. & Anderson, R.H. (2005). The morphological spectrum of ventricular noncompaction. *Cardiology in the Young*, Vol. 15, No. 4, (August 2005), pp. 345-364, ISSN 1047-9511

Jefferies, J.L. & Towbin, J.A. (2010). Dilated cardiomyopathy. *Lancet*, Vol. 375, No. 9716, (Febuary 27, 2010), pp. 752-762, ISSN 0140-6736

Gaita, F., Giustetto, C., Bianchi, F., Wolpert, C., Schimpf, R., Riccardi, R., Grossi, S., Richiardi, E. & Borggrefe, M. (2003). Short QT Syndrome: a familial cause of sudden death. *Circulation*, Vol. 108, No. 8, (August 18, 2003), pp. 965-970, ISSN 0009-7322

Kass, R.S. (2005). The channelopathies: novel insights into molecular and genetic mechanisms of human disease. *The Journal of Clinical Investigation*, Vol. 115, No. 8, (August), pp. 1986-1989, ISSN 0021-9738

Krittayaphong, R., Veerakul, G., Nademanee, K. & Kangkagate, C. (2003). Heart rate variability in patients with Brugada syndrome in Thailand. *European Heart Journal*, Vol. 24, No. 19, (October 2003), pp. 1771-1778, ISSN 0195-668x

Kushwaha, S.S., Fallon, J.T. & Fuster, V. (1997). Restrictive cardiomyopathy. *The New England Journal of Medicine*, Vol. 336, No. 4, (January 23, 1997), pp. 267-276, ISSN 0028-4793

Lowey, S. (2002). Functional consequences of mutations in the myosin heavy chain at sites implicated in familial hypertrophic cardiomyopathy. *Trends in Cardiovascular Medicine*, Vol. 12, No., 8, (November 2002), pp. 348-354, ISSN 1050-1738

Marcus, F.I., McKenna, W.J., Sherrill, D., Basso, C., Bauce, B., Bluemke, D.A., Calkins, H., Corrado, D., Cox, M.G., Daubert, J.P., Fontaine, G., Gear, K., Hauer, R., Nava, A., Picard, M.H., Protonotarios, N., Saffitz, J.E., Sanborn, D.M., Steinberg, J.S., Tandri,

H., Thiene, G., Towbin, J.A., Tsatsopoulou, A., Wichter, T. & Zareba, W. (2010). Diagnosis of arrhythmogenic right ventricular cardiomyopathy/dysplasia: proposed modification of the task force criteria. *Circulation*, Vol. 121, No. 13, (February 19, 2010), pp. 1533-1541, ISSN 0009-7322

Maron, B.J. (2002). Cardiology patient pages. Hypertrophic cardiomyopathy. *Circulation*, Vol. 106, No. 19, (November 2002), pp. 2419-2421, ISSN 0009-7322

Maron, B.J. (2008). The 2006 American Heart Association classification of cardiomyopathies is the gold standard. *Circulation Heart Failure*, Vol. 1, No. 1, (May 2008), pp. 72 75, ISSN 1941-3289

Maron, B.J., Towbin, J.A., Thiene, G., Antzelevitch, C., Corrado, D., Arnett, D., Moss, A.J., Seidman, C.E. & Young, J.B. (2006). Contemporary definitions and classification of the cardiomyopathies: an American Heart Association Scientific Statement from the Council on Clinical Cardiology, Heart Failure and Transplantation Committee; Quality of Care and Outcomes Research and Functional Genomics and Translational Biology Interdisciplinary Working Groups; and Council on Epidemiology and Prevention. *Circulation*, Vol. 113, No. 14, (March 27, 2006), pp. 1807-1816. ISSN 0009-7322

Modell, S.M. & Lehmann, M.H. (2006).The long QT syndrome family of cardiac ion channelopathies: a HuGE review. *Genetics in Medicine*, Vol. 8, No. 3, (March 2006), pp. 143-155, ISSN 1098-3600

Monserrat Iglesias, L. (2008). Left ventricular noncompaction: a disease in search of a definition. *Revista Espanola de Cardiologia*, Vol. 61, No. 2, (February 2008), pp. 112-115, ISSN 0300-8932

Nava, A., Bauce, B., Basso, C., Muriago, M., Rampazzo, A., Villanova, C., Daliento, L., Buja, G., Corrado, D., Danieli, G.A. & Thiene, G. (2000). Clinical profile and long-term follow-up of 37 families with arrhythmogenic right ventricular cardiomyopathy. *Journal of the American College of Cardiology*, Vol. 36, No. 7, (December 2000), pp. 2226-2233, ISSN 0735-1097

Parrillo, J.E. (2001). Inflammatory cardiomyopathy (myocarditis): which patients should be treated with anti-inflammatory therapy? *Circulation*, Vol. 104, No. 1, (July 3, 2001), pp. 4-6, ISSN 0009-7322

Protonotarios, N., Anastasakis, A., Antoniades, L., Chlouverakis, G., Syrris, P., Basso, C., Asimaki, A., Theopistou, A., Stefanadis, C., Thiene, G., McKenna, W.J. & Tsatsopoulou, A. (2011). Arrhythmogenic right ventricular cardiomyopathy/dysplasia on the basis of the revised diagnostic criteria in affected families with desmosomal mutations. *European Heart Journal*, Vol. 32, No. 9, (Febuary 22, 2011), pp. 1097-1104, ISSN 0195-668x

Richardson, P., McKenna, W., Bristow, M., Maisch, B., Mautner, B., O'Connell, J., Olsen, E., Thiene, G. & Goodwin, J. (1996). Report of the 1995 World Health Organization/International Society and Federation of Cardiology Task Force on the Definition and Classification of Cardiomyopathies. *Circulation*, Vol. 93, No. 5, (March 1, 1996), pp. 841-842, ISSN 0009-7322

Rosamond, W., Flegal, K., Furie, K., Go, A., Greenlund, K., Haase, N., Hailpern, S.M., Ho, M., Howard, V., Kissela, B., Kittner, S., Lloyd-Jones, D., McDermott, M., Meigs, J., Moy, C., Nichol, G., O'Donnell, C., Roger, V., Sorlie, P., Steinberger, J., Thom, T., Wilson, M. & Hong, Y. (2008). Heart disease and stroke statistics-2008 update: a report from the American Heart Association Statistics Committee and Stroke Statistics Subcommittee. *Circulation*, Vol. 117, No. 4, (January 29, 2008), pp. e25-e146, ISSN0009-7322

Schimpf, R., Wolpert, C., Gaita, F., Giustetto, C. & Borggrefe, M. (2005). Short QT syndrome. *Cardiovascular Research*, Vol. 67, No. 3, (August 15, 2005). pp. 357-366, ISSN 0008-6363

Sealove, B.A., Tiyyagura, S. & Fuster, V. (2008). Takotsubo cardiomyopathy. *Journal of General Internal Medicine*, Vol. 23, No. 11, (August 2008), pp. 1904-1908, ISSN 0884-8734

Selvetella, G. & Lembo, G. (2005). Mechanisms of cardiac hypertrophy. *Heart Failure Clinics*, Vol. 1, No. 2, (July 2005), pp. 263-273, ISSN 1551-7136

Sharkey, S.W., Lesser, J.R., Zenovich, A.G., Maron, M.S., Lindberg, J., Longe, T.F. & Maron, B.J. (2005). Acute and reversible cardiomyopathy provoked by stress in women from the United States. *Circulation*, Vol. 111, No. 4, (Febuary 1, 2005), pp. 472-479, ISSN 0009-7322

Taylor, M.R., Carniel, E. & Mestroni, L. (2006). Cardiomyopathy, familial dilated. *Orphanet Journal of Rare Diseases*, Vol. 1, (July13, 2006), pp. 27, ISSN 1750-1172

Thiene, G., Angelini, A., Basso, C., Calabrese, F. & Valente, M. (2000). The new definition and classification of cardiomyopathies. *Advances in Clinical Pathology*, Vol. 4, No. 2, (April, 2000), pp. 53-57, ISSN 1125-5552

Thiene, G., Corrado, D. & Basso, C. (2004). Cardiomyopathies: is it time for a molecular classification? *European Heart Journal*, Vol. 25, No. 20, (October 2004), 1772-1775, ISSN 0195-668x

Towbin, J.A., Lowe, A.M., Colan, S.D., Sleeper, L.A., Orav, E.J., Clunie, S., Messere, J., Cox, G.F., Lurie, P.R., Hsu, D., Canter, C., Wilkinson, J.D. & Lipshultz, S.E. (2006). Incidence, causes, and outcomes of dilated cardiomyopathy in children. *The Journal of the American Medical Association*, Vol. 296, No. 15, (October 18, 2006), pp. 1867-1876, ISSN 0098-7484

Wilde, A.A., Bhuiyan, Z.A., Crotti, L., Facchini, M., De Ferrari, G.M., Paul, T., Ferrandi, C., Koolbergen, D.R., Odero, A. & Schwartz, P.J. (2008). Left cardiac sympathetic denervation for catecholaminergic polymorphic ventricular tachycardia. *The New England Journal of Medicine*, Vol. 358, No. 19, (May 8, 2008), pp. 2024-2029, ISSN 0028-4793

2

Cardiomyopathy Detection from Electrocardiogram Features

Mirela Ovreiu and Dan Simon
Cleveland Clinic Foundation, Cleveland State University
United States

1. Introduction

Cardiomyopathy refers to diseases of the heart muscle that becomes enlarged, thick, or rigid. These changes affect the electrical stability of the myocardial cells, which predisposes the heart to failure or arrhythmias. Cardiomyopathy in its two common forms, dilated and hypertrophic, implies enlargement of the atria. Therefore, computer intelligence techniques are proposed for the recognition and classification of P wave features for cardiomyopathy diagnosis. The technique that we propose is a neuro-fuzzy network. The neuro-fuzzy classifier will be trained with innovative evolutionary algorithms, which have recently been shown to be efficient global optimizers.

Cardiomyopathy is a significant clinical problem which is mainly generated by volume/diastolic overload. To accommodate the increased blood volume, the heart chambers may stretch or dilate. Valvular regurgitation and congestive heart failure are two conditions that contribute to chamber dilation.

Cardiomyopathy is generally diagnosed by an electrocardiographic (ECG) investigation. In the current standards published by the American Heart Association, chamber hypertrophy or enlargement is a separate diagnostic category which can be detected with ECG analysis (Masson, Hancock, & Gettes, 2007). Although many algorithms have been implemented for ECG analysis, the proposed research is unique in several ways.

- We propose the development of **non-invasive** and **automatic cardiomyopathy diagnosis**, which has not been reported in the literature.
- We propose the development of algorithms for **P wave analysis**, which have not been reported in the literature.
- We propose the use of **5-lead ECG data**, which is more readily available than 12-lead data.
- We propose the use of a powerful **neuro-fuzzy architecture** for ECG analysis, which has not been reported in the literature.
- We propose neuro-fuzzy ECG classifier optimization using **evolutionary algorithms**, which has not been reported in the literature.

Our preliminary studies of postoperative cardiovascular patients reveal our hypothesis: the ECG presents different electrical activity for patients with cardiomyopathy, compared with patients who do not have cardiomyopathy. This working hypothesis indicates that an automated method that selects the best ECG parameters to include in a cardiomyopathy diagnosis algorithm will be extremely valuable. Although such a method will not be fool-proof or 100% correct, and thus cannot replace medical doctors, it will help physicians diagnose or prognose life threatening conditions such as stroke or ventricular or atrial fibrillation. This will expedite the initiation of medical treatment as appropriate to minimize the risk of these conditions, or to prevent their onsets.

Although it has long been suggested that cardiomyopathy is reflected in modification of ECG characteristics, statistics-based attempts to classify cardiomyopathy from the ECG have been underwhelming (Macfarlane, 2006; Magdic, Saul, 1997). Motivated by the universal approximation theorem for neuro-fuzzy networks discussed in the chapter, we hypothesize that earlier limitations may be overcome by a neuro-fuzzy classification model.

Cardiovascular diseases are the major cause of death in the western world, resulting in more than 800,000 deaths per year in the United States alone (American Heart Association, 2009). One in five Americans has some form of cardiovascular disease (Olson, 2004).

Cardiomyopathy is a significant clinical problem which is mainly generated by volume/diastolic overload. To accommodate the increased volume of blood, the heart chambers may stretch or dilate. Valvular regurgitation and congestive heart failure are two conditions that contribute to chamber dilation.

Cardiomyopathy is generally diagnosed by an echocardiograph investigation. For an echocardiography the patient has to be referred to a cardiologist or an echocardiographic investigation. But the electrocardiographic (ECG) investigation is always part of a cardiologic work-up.

The ECG represents the recording of the deflection of ionic current across myocardial cell membranes and throughout the extracellular space of the different tissues of the thoracic cavity. The ECG, in competition to many other techniques, retains an important role in diagnosis and prognosis of cardiovascular diseases.

It has been suggested that cardiomyopathy is reflected in modification of ECG characteristics such as P wave morphology. Previous statistics-based attempts to classify the cardiomyopathy from ECG have been underwhelming (Macfarlane, 2006; Magdic, Saul, 1997), but we hypothesize that these limitations can be overcome using a hybrid neuro-fuzzy classification model. To test this hypothesis and direct the results to patient care, we follow these directions. First we design a neuro-fuzzy model to diagnose cardiomyopathy. Then we train the network using an aquired clinical database of ECG signals.

Neuro-fuzzy systems can be trained with derivative-based methods like gradient descent (Chen, Linkens, 2001; Linkens, Chen, 1999) or with evolutionary algorithms such as genetic algorithms and swarm intelligence (Kennedy, Eberhart, & Shi, 2001). Evolutionary algorithms have the advantage of not requiring derivative information, and have less likelihood of getting stuck in a local optimum. Hence we use a new biologically motivated optimization algorithm called biogeography-based optimization (BBO) (Simon, 2008) to train the neuro-fuzzy ECG classification network. We also incorporate opposition-based learning in the BBO algorithm (Ergezer, Simon, & Du, 2009) for better classification.

2. Background

2.1 Cardiomyopathy

The term "cardiomyopathy" defines a group of diseases primarily affecting the cardiac muscle by weakening it or changing its structure. Cardiomyopathy can be acquired or inherited, and in many cases its cause is unknown. Hypertrophic cardiomyopathy is inherited and is supposed to be a result of defects of genes that regulate heart muscle growth. Abnormal cardiac enlargement can be due to an increase in length or diameter of existing cardiac muscle cells (Olson, 2004). Cardiomyopathy, through electrical instability of myocardial cells, is associated with cardiac conduction abnormalities that can degenerate to arrhythmia or heart failure (Dische, 1972).

Cardiomyopathies, especially hypertrophic, are considered a common cause of sudden cardiac death in young adults and children (Ingles, Semsarian, 2007; Bar-Cohen, Silka, 2008). The Chagas and idiopathic dilated etiologies of cardiomyopathy led to Pereira et al.'s study in adults (Pereira et al., 2010); after 40 months, almost half of the cases studied (113 out of 284) registered deaths (104) or heart transplants (9).

The ECG records the deflection of ionic current across myocardial cell membranes and through the extracellular space of the thoracic cavity tissues. The history of cardiomyopathy research reveals the evolution of the analysis of ECG correlations. Due to the left ventricle's critical role, initial studies were focused only on the ECG features of the hypertrophic left ventricle (Sox, Garber, Littenberg, 1989). The QRS and T waves, as the reflections of ventricular depolarization and repolarization respectively, were analyzed (Ziegler, 1970). In the study by Sox et al., citing the Framingham Study, the left ventricular hypertrophy (LVH) was defined by a prolonged ventricular activation period of 0.05 s, tall R waves, depressed ST segments, and inverted T waves (Sox, Garber, Littenberg, 1989). Ziegler was the first to analyze T waves related to LVH; he presented different patterns of the QRS and T configurations into left or right precordial limb leads (Ziegler, 1970). The P wave portrays atrial electrical activity, so changes in the atrial action potential and substrate are reflected in P wave timing or morphology (Chandy, 2004). Bahl et al. presented the P wave changes associated with the type and stage of the disease (Bahl, 1972). Analyzing the four chamber enlargements, Johnson et al. presented P wave changes for enlarged left and right atria (Johnson, Horan, & Flowers, 1977).

The atria, characterized by thin walls, respond to volume and pressure overload due to dilatation. Moreover, the enlargement of the associated ventricle is recognized as the cause of the enlargement of the atrium (Macfarlane, 2006; Magdic, Saul, 1997). The right atrium enlargement is recognized by the increased amplitude of the P wave (0.25 mV) while left atrial abnormality is reflected by the lengthened P wave duration (>120 ms) as well as a notched P wave.

The American Heart Association, American College of Cardiology Foundation, and the Heart Rhythm Society, recently concluded on standards to be used when interpreting ECG data related to cardiomyopathy (Hancock et al., 2009). In left ventricular hypertrophy, the P wave shape is mentioned as a criterion. In right ventricular hypertrophy (LVH), a P wave amplitude larger than 0.25 mV in lead II is presented as a threshold. Left atrial abnormality implies a prolongation of the total atrial activation time (>120 ms), widely notched P wave, and possible changes in P wave area. The right atrial abnormality list includes a larger amplitude of the P wave (> 0.25 mV) and a prolongation of the P wave in patients after cardiac surgery, which is the case for the patients in our proposed research.

Our proposed algorithm presents the advantage of compatibility with the clinical Cardio-Vascular Intensive Care Unit (CVICU) setting since it is designed to analyze P wave parameters from a 5-lead ECG, versus the laboratory 12-lead ECG. P wave delineation is made automatically on the ECG signal using wavelet transforms. The P wave features obtained by the wavelets are then processed by a neuro-fuzzy system. Neuro-fuzzy systems are combinations of fuzzy systems and artificial neural networks. Such combined systems have the advantage that they can learn faster and more accurately than an individual artificial neural network or fuzzy logic system. A benefit over artificial neural networks is that the rules that describe the system are explicit, thus permitting easy interpretation and validation.

Considering the frequent association of cardiomyopathy and atrial fibrillation, a future application of this successful classification process is the inclusion of the results in an automatic prediction algorithm for atrial fibrillation (AF). AF is a threatening arrhythmia that is encountered in 25% of post-cardiovascular surgical patients in the CVICU of the Cleveland Clinic.

Cardiomyopathy diagnosis will be performed by a multivariate, neuro-fuzzy classification model that uses P wave parameters to generate a cardiomyopathy classification index. Artificial Neural Networks are universal approximators (Buckley, Hayashi, 1995), and there has also been extensive work to prove that neuro-fuzzy systems can approximate any continuous function to any desired degree of accuracy (Feuring, Lippe, 1999). Alvisi et al. (Alvisi et al., 2006) have studied the performances of fuzzy logic and Artificial Neural Networks, revealing the weaknesses and strengths of each of the methods. The strengths can be emphasized, and some of the weaknesses can be attenuated, by combining the techniques into a hybrid neuro-fuzzy model. **The universal approximation theorem is the reason that a neuro-fuzzy system may be able to overcome the limitations of previous statistics-based methods for ECG analysis.**

2.2 Neuro-fuzzy networks

Consider a multi-input, single-output fuzzy logic system. Our discussion can be easily generalized to multiple output systems, but restricting our discussion to single-output systems simplifies the notation considerably. In addition, the ECG classification system that we consider in this paper is single-output. The ith rule R_i of the fuzzy system can be written as follows (Chen, Linkens, 2001).

$$R_i : \text{If } x_1 \text{ is } A_{i1} \text{ and } \dots \text{ and } x_m \text{ is } A_{im} \text{ then}$$
$$y = z_i(x), \qquad (i = 1, \cdots, p). \tag{1}$$

The inputs x_i and the output y are linguistic variables, A_{ij} are fuzzy sets, and $z_i(x)$ is a function of the input $x = [x_1 \dots x_m]^T$. The output function $z_i(x)$ typically takes one of the following forms: (1) singleton, (2) fuzzy set, (3) linear function. If the fuzzy system uses center average defuzzification, product inference, and singleton fuzzification, then $z_i(x) = z_i$ (a singleton) and the fuzzy system output can be written as

$$y = \frac{\sum_{i=1}^{p} z_i \prod_{j=1}^{m} \mu_{ij}(x_j)}{\sum_{i=1}^{p} \prod_{j=1}^{m} \mu_{ij}(x_j)} \tag{2}$$

where $\mu_{ij}(x_{ij})$ denotes the degree of membership of x_j in R_i. As in many neuro-fuzzy networks, we use a Gaussian form for μ_{ij}:

$$\mu_{ij}(x_j) = \exp\left(\frac{-(x_j - c_{ij})^2}{\sigma_{ij}^2}\right) \tag{3}$$

where c_{ij} is the jth element of the center of the ith rule, and σ_{ij} is its standard deviation. In this case, Eq. (2) becomes

$$y = \frac{w}{\sum_{i=1}^{p} m_i(x)} \tag{4}$$

$$w = \sum_{i=1}^{p} z_i m_i(x) \tag{5}$$

$$m_i(x) = exp[-(x - c_i)^T P^{-2}(x - c_i)] \tag{6}$$

where $c_i = [c_{i1} \cdots c_{im}]^T$ and $P = \text{diag}(\sigma_1, \cdots, \sigma_m)$. Eq. (5) is in the form of a radial basis function, which is a type of neural network (Chen, Linkens, 2001). The system of Eqs. (5) and (6) is therefore called a neuro-fuzzy system. It can be depicted as shown in Figure 1.

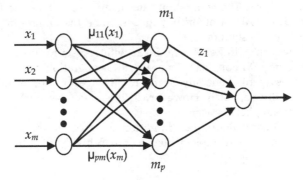

Fig. 1. Multi-input single-output neuro-fuzzy system architecture

The neuro-fuzzy system in Figure 1 is a function of the pxm elements of the membership centers c_{ij}, the pxm elements of the membership standard deviations σ_{ij}, and the p elements of the singleton outputs z_i. There are thus $p(2m+1)$ parameters that define the neuro-fuzzy system. For a given neuro-fuzzy system architecture and a given training set of input/output data, the neuro-fuzzy system parameters can be optimized with respect to these $p(2m+1)$ parameters.

2.3 Biogeography-Based Optimization (BBO)

Biogeography-based optimization (BBO) is a recently-developed population-based evolutionary optimization algorithm (Simon, 2008). As its name implies, BBO is motivated by biogeography, which is the study of the distribution of species over time and space (Whittaker, 1998). BBO has demonstrated good performance on various benchmark functions (Lomolino, Riddle, & Brown, 2009; Simon, 2008). It has also been successfully applied to several real-world optimization problems, including sensor selection (Simon, 2008), power system optimization (Rarick et al., 2009), groundwater detection (Kundra, Kaur, & Panchal, 2009), and satellite image classification (Panchal et al., 2009).

Given an optimization problem and a population of candidate solutions (individuals), a biogeography-based optimization (BBO) solution with high fitness is likely to share its features with other solutions, and a solution with low fitness is unlikely to share its features. Conversely, a solution with high fitness is unlikely to accept features from other solutions, while a solution low fitness is likely to accept features. Solution feature sharing, which is called immigration and emigration, tends to improve the solutions and thus evolve a good solution to the problem.

In biogeography-based optimization (BBO), each individual solution has its own immigration rate λ_i and emigration rate μ_i. A good solution has relatively high μ and low λ, while the converse is true for a poor solution. The immigration rate and the emigration rate are functions of the fitness of the solution. They are often calculated as

$$\lambda_i = f_i/n$$
$$\mu_i = 1 - \lambda_i \tag{7}$$

where n is the population size and f_i is the fitness rank of the ith individual (the most fit individual has a rank $f_i = 1$). The immigration rates λ_i are interpreted by the BBO algorithm as immigration probabilities. The emigration rates μ_i are proportional to fitness and so are used in a roulette-wheel type of algorithm to determine the emigrating solution in case immigration is selected for a solution.

Although the migration rates in Eq. (1) are linear with respect to fitness rank as originally proposed in earlier study (Simon, 2008), more natural migration rates which are sigmoid with respect to fitness rank generally seem to give better optimization performance (Lomolino, Riddle, & Brown, 2009). However, in this paper we retain the original linear migration rates for the simplicity reason.

As with other evolutionary algorithms, mutation is typically implemented to increase exploration, and elitism is often implemented to retain highly fit solutions. The standard BBO algorithm is shown in Figure 2.

For each solution H_i
    For each solution feature s
        Select solution H_i with probability proportional to λ_i
        If solution H_i is selected then
            Select H_j with probability proportional to μ_j
            If H_j is selected then
                $H_i(s) \leftarrow H_j(s)$
            end
        end
    next solution feature
    Probabilistically mutate H_i
next solution

Fig. 2. One generation of the standard BBO algorithm.

2.4 Oppositional BBO

Opposition-based learning (OBL) has been introduced as a method that can be used by Evolutionary Algorithms (EAs) to accelerate convergence speed by comparing the fitness of an individual to its opposite and retaining the fitter one in the population (Rahnamayan, Tizhoosh, & Salama, 2007; Tizhoosh, 2005). The "opposite" of an individual is defined as the reflection of that individual's features across the midpoint of the search space. Opposition-based differential evolution (ODE) (Rahnamayan, Tizhoosh, & Salama, 2008.) was the first application of OBL to Evolutionary Algorithms (EAs). OBL was first incorporated in BBO in earlier research study (Ergezer, Simon, & Du, 2009) and was shown to improve BBO by a significant amount on standard optimization benchmarks.

Given an Evolutionary Algorithm (EA) population member x, there are at least three different types of oppositional points that can be defined. These oppositional points are referred to as the opposite x_o, the quasi-opposite x_q, and the quasi-reflected-opposite x_r. Figure 3 illustrates these points for an arbitrary x in a one-dimensional domain. The point c is the center of the domain, x_o the reflection of x across c, x_q is a randomly generated point from a uniform distribution between c and x_o, and x_r is a randomly generated point from a uniform distribution between x and c.

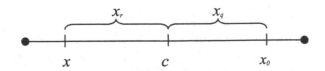

Fig. 3. Illustration of an arbitrary EA individual x, its opposite x_o, its quasi-opposite x_q, and its quasi-reflected-opposite x_r, in a one-dimensional domain.

OBL is essentially a more intelligent way of implementing exploration instead of generating random mutations. Another way of viewing OBL is from the perspective of social revolutions in human society. Society often progresses on the basis of a few individuals who embrace philosophies that are not just random, but that are deliberately contrary to accepted norms. Given that an EA individual is described by the vector x, and that the solution to the optimization problem is uniformly distributed in the search domain, it is shown in Rahnamayan' study (Rahnamayan, Tizhoosh, Salama, 2007) that x_q is probably closer to the solution than x or x_o. Further, it is presented in our earlier publication (Ergezer, Simon, & Du, 2009) that x_r is probably closer to the solution than x_q. These results are nonintuitive, but results related to random numbers are often nonintuitive, and the OBL results are derived not only analytically by also using simulation.

In this paper we use oppositional BBO (OBBO) to train the neuro-fuzzy ECG classification network. Suppose that the population size is N. OBBO works by generating a population of N opposite individuals which are the opposite of the current population. Then, given the entire $2N$ individuals comprised of both the original and the opposite populations, the best N individuals are retained for the next population. However, this does not occur at each generation. Instead it occurs randomly with a probability of J_r at each generation. J_r is called the jump rate. Based on (Rahnamayan, Tizhoosh, & Salama, 2006) we use $J_r = 0.3$ in this paper. In order to increase the likelihood of improvement at each generation we implement OBBO as follows. At each generation, we save the original population of N individuals before creating a population of N new individuals via migration. We then create an opposite population of N additional individuals if indicated by the jump rate. Of the total $2N$ or $3N$ individuals, we finally select the best N for the next generation. Note that this approach guarantees that the best individual in each generation is at least as good as that of the previous generation. This is similar to a $(\mu+\lambda)$ evolutionary strategy (Du, Simon, & Ergezer, 2009), whose parameters are not to be confused with the μ and λ migration parameters in BBO. The resulting OBBO algorithm is summarized in Figure 4.

$H^{(1)} \leftarrow H$ (make a copy of the population H)
For each solution $H_i \in H^{(1)}$ ($i = 1, ..., N$)
    For each solution feature s
        Select solution H_i with probability proportional to λ_i
        If solution H_i is selected then
            Select H_j with probability proportional to μ_j
            If H_j is selected then
                $H_i(s) \leftarrow H_j^{(1)}$
            end
        end
        next solution feature
        Probabilistically mutate H_i
    next solution
    if rand(0,1) $< J_r$ then
        Use H to create an N-member opposite population $H^{(2)}$
    else
        $H^{(2)} = \varnothing$
    end
    Copy the best N individuals from $\{H, H^{(1)}, H^{(2)}\}$ to H

Fig. 4. One generation of oppositional BBO (OBBO).

3. ECG data

In preparation for the testing of a cardiomyopathy diagnosis model, a database of long-duration ECG signals was collected. The database includes signals from 55 subjects, 18 of them with cardiomyopathy. Not all subjects experienced chronic or paroxysmal atrial fibrillation. The cardiomyopathy group contained 10 males and 8 females with a mean age of 54 (range 23–88) years. The control group contained 22 males and 15 females with a mean age of 60 (range 27–77) yrs. The inclusion criteria were the same for both groups: no chronic or paroxystic atrial fibrillation and no perioperative pacing.

ECG parameters describing P wave morphology were computed for each minute of data recording for all 55 patients in the training data set. This set of ECG parameter values constitutes the input component of the training data set for neuro-fuzzy model development. For additional details of ECG parameter computation algorithms see (Bashour et al., 2004; Visinescu et al., 2004; Visinescu, 2005; Visinescu et al., 2006; Ovreiu et al., 2008)

The P wave from the electrocardiogram reflects the electrical activity of the atria and may indicate the existence of irregularities in electrical conduction. Using a previously developed P wave detection method, the starting, ending, and maximum points of the P wave were determined (Visinescu, 2005). The average P wave morphology parameters were computed once per minute. The P wave morphology parameters included the following:

a. Duration
b. Amplitude
c. A shape parameter which represents monophasicity or biphasicity
d. Inflection point, which is the duration of the P wave between the onset and the peak points
e. Energy ratio, defined as the fraction between the right atrial excitation energy and the total atrial excitation energy.

Initial investigation revealed that the monophasicity / biphasicity parameter did not vary appreciably between cardiomyopathy and control patients. We therefore discarded the monophasicity / biphasicity parameter from our data set. Differences between the remaining P wave morphology parameters for cardiomyopathy and control patients in the training database are presented in Figure 5. Based on the standard deviation bars, there is apparently important information included in these parameters. Their usefulness in identifying the patients with cardiomyopathy is determined by the proposed neuro-fuzzy model as discussed in the following section.

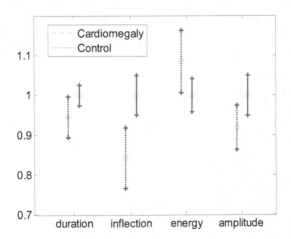

Fig. 5. P wave characteristics of cardiomyopathy and control patients. Data are normalized to the mean values of the control patients. Error bars show one standard deviation.

4. Experimental results

4.1 Problem setup

Cardiomyopathy diagnosis is performed by a multivariate, neuro-fuzzy classification model that uses current values of ECG P wave parameters to generate a cardiomyopathy classification index. The initial model is a multi-input single-output fuzzy inference system with a three-layer architecture (Figure 1). The fuzzification layer takes crisp parameter values and determines their memberships in linguistic categories (low, medium, high, etc.).

Each of these fuzzy variables are then input to each node of the fuzzy rule layer (i.e., the middle layer shown in Figure 1). The model output, which is the cardiomyopathy classification index, is the weighted average of the output rules.

Since we have four inputs (see Figure 5), we have $m = 4$ in Figure 1. The number of middle-layer neurons is equal to p and should be chosen as a tradeoff between good training performance and good generalization. If p is too small then training performance will be poor because we will not have enough degrees of freedom in the neuro-fuzzy network. If p is too large then test performance will be poor because the training algorithm will tend to "memorize" the training inputs rather than obtaining a good generalization for test data.

The output y shown in Eq. (4) is chosen to be +1 for cardiomyopathy patients and –1 for control patients. The ECG database is used for training and the output of the neuro-fuzzy system is compared to the known classification of the ECG patient. The RMS training error is defined as

$$E = \sqrt{\frac{1}{N}\sum_{i=1}^{N}(d_i - y_i)^2} \tag{8}$$

where N is the number of training inputs, d_i is the desired output of the ith training datum (+1 or –1), and y_i is the corresponding neuro-fuzzy output. In order to determine the best value of p (the number of middle-layer neurons) we run 10 Monte Carlo simulations with various values for p and compare training and testing errors. The BBO parameters that we use are as follows:

- Population size = 200
- Mutation rate = 2% per solution feature
- Generation limit = 50

Mutation is implemented by randomly generating a new parameter from a uniform distribution between the minimum and maximum parameter bounds. The parameter bounds that we use are as follows:

- Output singletons $z_i \in [-10, +10]$
- Membership centroids $c_{ij} \in [0, \pi]$
- Membership standard deviations $\sigma_{ij} \in [0.01, 5]$

We use ECG data from 55 test subjects as described in Section 3, which includes 37 control patients and 18 cardiomyopathy patients. We randomly divide the patients into approximately equal numbers of training patients and test patients. We therefore have 9 cardiomyopathy patients and 19 control patients for training the network, and 9 cardiomyopathy patients and 18 control patients for testing the network. We randomly choose 200 ECG data points from a 700-minute time interval for each patient for both training and testing. Therefore, we have 200×(9+19) = 5600 data points for training, and 200×(9+18) = 5400 data points for testing.

4.2 Parameter tuning and results

Table 1 shows the minimum training error attained as specified in Eq. (2) for various numbers of middle-layer neurons, along with the resulting correct classification rate for training and testing. An ECG data point is classified as cardiomyopathy if the neuro-fuzzy output $y > 0$, and control if the neuro-fuzzy output $y < 0$. The quantity of primary interest is the correct classification rate for the test data, and Table 1 shows that this is attained with 3 middle-layer neurons. Fewer neurons gives too few degrees of freedom, and more neurons results in a tendency of the neuro-fuzzy system to overfit the training data and hence not provide adequate generalization for the test data.

p	Training Error		Train CCR (%)		Test CCR (%)	
	Best	Mean	Best	Mean	Best	Mean
2	0.85	0.88	76	72	66	58
3	0.77	0.84	82	77	75	62
4	0.78	0.83	84	77	65	55
5	0.78	0.83	82	76	63	58

Table 1. Training error and correct classification rate (CCR) for training and testing as a function of the number of middle layer neurons p.

Next we implement OBBO to explore the effect of OBL on classification performance. Table 2 shows results for three different OBL options: standard BBO, OBBO using quasi-opposition (Q-BBO), and OBBO using quasi-reflected opposition (R-BBO). We use the same population size, mutation rate, and generation limit as discussed earlier. We use 3 middle-layer neurons as indicated by Table 1. Table 2 shows that OBBO using quasi-opposition provides the best neuro-fuzzy classification performance when test performance is used as the criterion.

Note that the numbers in Tables 1 and 2 do not match exactly because they are the results of different sets of Monte Carlo simulations. In future work we will use a more extensive set of simulations in order to obtain results with a smaller margin of error.

	Training Error		Train CCR (%)		Test CCR (%)	
	Best	Mean	Best	Mean	Best	Mean
BBO	0.77	0.86	84	76	66	58
Q-BBO	0.83	0.86	79	74	69	62
R-BBO	0.80	0.85	81	75	65	60

Table 2. Training error and correct classification rate (CCR) for training and testing for alternative implementations oppositional BBO.

After settling on Q-BBO with 3 middle-layer neurons, we explore the effect of mutation rate on Q-BBO performance. Table 3 shows neuro-fuzzy results for various mutation rates. We use the same population size and generation limit as before. Table 3 shows that mutation rate does not have a strong effect on neuro-fuzzy system results, but based on test data performance, a low mutation rate generally gives better results than a high mutation rate.

Mutation rate	Training Error		Train CCR (%)		Test CCR (%)	
(%)	Best	Mean	Best	Mean	Best	Mean
0.1	0.79	0.85	81	76	71	61
0.2	0.82	0.86	80	75	72	59
0.5	0.77	0.85	82	76	69	62
1.0	0.80	0.85	80	74	67	57
2.0	0.83	0.86	79	74	69	62
5.0	0.82	0.87	81	74	68	58
10.0	0.80	0.87	78	73	65	59

Table 3. Training error and correct classification rate (CCR) for different mutation rates using Q-BBO.

Figure 6 shows the progress for a typical Q-BBO training simulation. Note that the minimum training error in the top plot is monotonically nonincreasing due to the inherent elitism of the algorithm (see Figure 3). However, the average cost in the top plot, along with the success rates in the bottom plot, sometimes increases and sometimes decreases from one generation to the next. The results shown in Figure 6 also indicate that better results might be obtained if the generation limit were increased. However, care must be taken when increasing the generation limit. As the generation count increases, the training error will continue to decrease but the test error will eventually begin to increase due to overtraining (Tetko, Livingstone,& Luik, 1995).

The Q-BBO training run illustrated in Figure 6 resulted in the following neuro-fuzzy parameters:

$$c = \begin{bmatrix} 0.513 & 0.116 & 0.981 & 0.065 \\ 0.316 & 0.930 & 0.138 & 0.214 \\ 0.899 & 0.235 & 0.041 & 0.613 \end{bmatrix} \tag{9}$$

$$\sigma = \begin{bmatrix} 1.119 & 0.409 & 0.133 & 0.101 \\ 0.326 & 0.805 & 1.963 & 1.529 \\ 1.825 & 0.356 & 0.858 & 0.438 \end{bmatrix} \tag{10}$$

$$z = \begin{bmatrix} 1.641 & -0.967 & 0.779 \end{bmatrix}. \tag{11}$$

Recall that we used a c range of $[0, \pi]$, but from Eq. (3) the highest membership centroid was less than 1 after Q-BBO training. This indicates that we could decrease the c range in order to get better resolution during training.

Similarly, recall that we used a σ range of $[0.01, 5]$, but from Eq. (4) the highest standard deviation was less than 2 after Q-BBO training. This indicates that we could decrease the σ range in order to get better resolution during training.

Finally, recall that we used an output singleton z range of $[-10, +10]$, but from Eq. (5) the output singletons were between -1 and 2 after Q-BBO training. This indicates that we could decrease the z range in order to get better resolution during training.

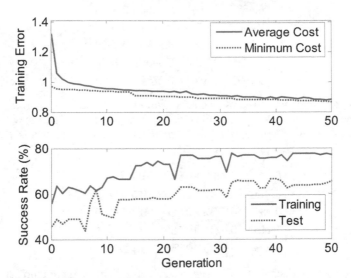

Fig. 6. Typical Q-BBO training results.

4.3 Clustering and pruning

The appropriate number of clusters in the neuro-fuzzy system is equivalent to the number of middle-layer neurons p shown in Figure 1. Determination of the optimal number of fuzzy rules is equivalent to finding a suitable number of clusters for the given data set. This can also be performed using fuzzy c-means clustering (Chen, Linkens, 2001; Linkens, Chen, 1999). Clustering is itself a multiobjective optimization problem that maximizes compactness within clusters, maximizes separation between clusters, and maximizes neuro-fuzzy system performance.

In the previous section we solved for cluster count using a direct approach involving manual tuning (see Table 1). However, we could also solve for cluster count by observing the output singletons z_i after training, discarding those that are significantly smaller than the others, and then retraining the network. This is a type of pruning. For example, when using BBO to train the neuro-fuzzy system with 5 middle-layer neurons, a typical result for the output singletons after convergence is

$$z = [1.766 \quad 1.880 \quad -1.712 \quad 0.392 \quad -1.542].$$

It is seen that the magnitude of z_4 (0.392) is smaller by a factor of 4 than any of the other elements of z. This indicates that the corresponding fuzzy rule might be able to be safely removed from the neuro-fuzzy system without sacrificing performance. Retuning should then be performed because the neuro-fuzzy parameters will need to be adjusted to compensate for the network size reduction.

Another way to check if we are using too many middle-layer neurons is by looking at the distance between fuzzy membership function centers. If, after training, two membership function centers are very close to each other, that indicates that those two fuzzy sets could be combined. For example, the matrix of fuzzy centroids after a typical training run with 5 middle-layer neurons (i.e., 5 fuzzy membership sets) is given by

$$c = \begin{bmatrix} 0.5587 & 0.0046 & 0.9480 & 0.6628 \\ 0.4908 & 0.3719 & 0.4274 & 0.2847 \\ 0.5534 & 0.9005 & 0.9880 & 0.2659 \\ 0.9839 & 0.7428 & 0.3904 & 0.2067 \\ 0.9992 & 0.6061 & 0.2754 & 0.2185 \end{bmatrix}.$$

Each row of c corresponds to a fuzzy set centroid, and each column of c corresponds to one dimension of the input data. A cursory look at the c matrix shows that rows 4 and 5 are similar to each other. A matrix of Euclidean distances between centroids (i.e., between columns of c) can be derived as

$$\Delta c = \begin{bmatrix} 0 & 0.7439 & 0.9807 & 1.1157 & 1.0980 \\ 0.7439 & 0 & 0.7732 & 0.6231 & 0.5838 \\ 0.9807 & 0.7732 & 0 & 0.7556 & 0.8919 \\ 1.1157 & 0.6231 & 0.7556 & 0 & 0.1797 \\ 1.0980 & 0.5838 & 0.7556 & 0.1797 & 0 \end{bmatrix}$$

where Δc_{ij} is the Euclidean distance between centroids i and j. The Δc matrix indicates that fuzzy centroids 4 and 5 are much closer to each other than the other centroids, which implies that the corresponding membership functions overlap, and so they could be combined. Afterward, the neuro-fuzzy system should be retrained to compensate for the change in its structure.

4.4 Fine tuning using gradient information
The BBO algorithm that we used, like other Evolutionary Algorithms (EAs), does not depend on gradient information. Therein lies its strength relative to gradient-based optimization methods. Evolutionary Algorithms (EAs) can be used for global optimization since they do not rely on local gradient information. Since the neuro-fuzzy system shown in Figure 1 may have multiple optima, BBO training is less likely to get stuck in a local optima compared to gradient-based optimization.

However, additional performance improvement could be obtained in the neuro-fuzzy classifier by using gradient information in conjunction with EA-based optimization. Gradient-based methods can be combined with EAs in order to take advantage of the strengths of each method. First we can use BBO, as above, in order to find neuro-fuzzy parameters that are in the neighborhood of the global optimum. Then we can use a gradient-based method to fine tune the BBO result. The most commonly-used gradient-based method is gradient descent clustering (Chen, Linkens, 2001; Linkens, Chen, 1999). Gradient descent can be further improved by using an adaptive learning rate and momentum term (Nauck, Klawonn, Kruse, 1997).

Kalman filtering is a gradient-based method that can give better fuzzy system and neural network training results than gradient descent (Simon, 2002a, 2002b). Constrained Kalman filtering can further improve fuzzy system results by optimally constraining the network parameters (Simon, 2002c). H-infinity estimation is another gradient-based method that can be used for fuzzy system training to improve robustness to data errors (Simon, 2005).

4.5 Training criterion
The ultimate goal of the neuro-fuzzy network is to maximize correct classification percentage. If the neuro-fuzzy output is greater than 0, then the ECG is classified as cardiomyopathy;

otherwise, the ECG is classified as non-cardiomyopathy. The bottom plot in Figure 6 shows that while RMS training error is monotonically nondecreasing, the success rate for the training data is non-monotonic. We could more directly address the problem of ECG data classification by using classification success rate as our fitness function rather than trying to minimize the RMS error of Eq. (2). That is, in fact, one of the advantages of EA training relative to gradient-based methods – the fitness function does not have to be differentiable. However, if we use classification success rate as our fitness function, and then try to use a gradient-based method for fine-tuning, the cost functions of the two training methods would be inconsistent.

5. Conclusion

We have shown that clinical ECG data can be correctly classified as cardiomyopathy or non-cardiomyopathy using a neuro-fuzzy network training by biogeography-based optimization (BBO). Our results show a correct classification rate on test data of over 60%. Better results can undoubtedly be attained with further training, but the main goal of this initial research was to demonstrate feasibility and to establish a framework for further refinement.

Although our preliminary results are good, there are many enhancements that need to be made in order to improve performance and incorporate this work into a commercial product. For example, demographic information needs to be included with the ECG data. Some of the test ECGs were correctly classified 100% of the time, while others had a very low success rate. Figure 7 shows the classification success rate for the test data as a function of patient ID. Some patients generated ECG data that was successfully classified as cardiomyopathy / non-cardiomyopathy only 2% of the time, while others generated data that was successfully classified 100% of the time. This indicates that demographic data is important and that we should group patients into similar groups for testing and training. Some of these data include gender, race, medication usage, and age. This will become feasible as we perform more clinical studies and collect data from more patients.

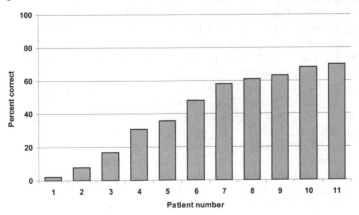

Fig. 7. ECG classification success rate for test patients.

We note that our results are based on snapshots of the data at single instants of time. We could presumably get better results by using a "majority rules" strategy for data collected over several minutes. For example, suppose that test accuracy is 60% for a given patient. We could use ECG data at three separate time instants and diagnose cardiomyopathy if the neuro-fuzzy network predicts cardiomyopathy for two or more of the data. This would boost test accuracy from 60% to 65%, assuming that the probability of correct classification is independent from one time instant to the next. We could then further improve accuracy by using more time instants.

A strong reason for investigating this cardiac anomaly is its association to Atrial Fibrillation occurrence. The availability of ECG registrations and efficiency in time and cost savings of such a different approach, especially in cardiovascular surgical patients would imply as a future work, the inclusion of this automated classification algorithm into a bed side monitor indicator that might be used in future classification and/or forecasting algorithms under investigation.

6. Acknowledgement

This work was partially supported by Grant 0826124 in the CMMI Division of the Engineering Directorate of the National Science Foundation and Grant NCRP 10CRP2600305 from American Heart Association.

7. References

Alvisi, S., Mascellani, G., Franchini, M., & Bardossy, A. (2006) – Water level forecasting through fuzzy logic and artificial neural network approaches, *Hydrology and Earth System Sciences*, 10 (1), pp. 1-17, 2006

American Heart Association, (2009). *Heart Disease and Stroke Statistics – 2009 Update*, www.americanheart.org/ presenter.jhtml?identifier=3018163

Bahl, O. (1972) – Electrocardiographic and vectorcardiographic pattern in cardiomyopathy, *Cardiovascular Clinics*, 4 (1), pp. 95-112, 1972

Bar-Cohen, Y., Silka, M. (2008) – Sudden cardiac death in pediatrics, *Current Opinion in Pediatrics*, 20 (5), pp. 517-521, 2008

Bashour, C., Visinescu, M., Gopakumaran, B., Wazni, O., Carragio, F., Yared, J., & Starr, N. (2004). Characterization of premature atrial contraction activity prior to the onset of postoperative atrial fibrillation in cardiac surgery patients, *Chest*, 126, 4 (2004), 831S.

Buckley, J. and Hayashi, Y. (1995) – Neural Nets for Fuzzy Systems, *Fuzzy Sets and Systems*, 71 (3), pp. 265-276, 1995

Chandy, J., Nakai, T., Lee, R., Bellows, W., Dzankic, S., & Leung, J. (2004) – Increases in P-wave Dispersion Predict Postoperative Atrial Fibrillation After Coronary Artery Bypass Graft Surgery, *Anesthesia & Analgesia*, 98, pp. 303-310, 2004

Chen, M. and Linkens, D. (2001). A systematic neuro-fuzzy modelling framework with application to material property prediction, *IEEE Transactions on Systems, Man, and Cybernetics – Part B: Cybernetics*, 31, 5 (2001), pp. 781-790.

Dische, M. R. (1972) – Observations on the morphological changes of the developing heart. *Cardiovascular Clinics*, 4 (3), pp. 175-191, 1972

Du, D., Simon, D., & Ergezer, M. (2009). Biogeography-based optimization combined with evolutionary strategy and immigration refusal. *In Proceedings of the IEEE Conference on Systems, Man, and Cybernetics (San Antonio, Texas, October 2009)*. pp. 1023–1028.

Ergezer, M., Simon D., & Du, D. (2009). Oppositional biogeography-based optimization. *In Proceedings of the IEEE Conference on Systems, Man, and Cybernetics (San Antonio, Texas, October 2009)*. pp. 1035–1040.

Feuring, T. and Lippe, W.-M. (1999) – The fuzzy neural network approximation lemma, *Fuzzy Sets and Systems*, 102 (2), pp. 227-236, 1999

Hancock, E.W., Mirvis, D.M., Okin, P., et al (2009) – AHA/ACCF/HRS recommendations for the standardization of interpretation of the electrocardiogram: part V: electrocardiogram changes associated with cardiac chamber hypertrophy: a scientific statement from the American Heart Association, Council on Clinical Cardiology; The American College of Cardiology Foundation, and the Heart Rhythm Society, *Journal of American College of Cardiology*, 53: pp. 992-1002, 2009

Heart Disease and Stroke Statistics,
    http://www.americanheart.org/presenter.jhtml?identifier=3018163, 2010

Ingles, J, Semsarian, C (2007) – Sudden cardiac death in the young: A clinical genetic approach, *Internal Medicine Journal*, 37 (1), pp. 32-37, 2007

Johnson, J. C., Horan, L. G., & Flowers, N. C. (1977) – Diagnostic accuracy of the electrocardiogram, *Cardiovascular Clinics*, 8 (3), pp. 25-40, 1977

Kennedy, J., Eberhart, R., & Shi, Y. (2001). *Swarm Intelligence*. Morgan Kaufmann,.

Kundra, H., Kaur, A., & Panchal, V. (2009). An integrated approach to biogeography based optimization with case based reasoning for retrieving groundwater possibility. In *Proceedings of the 8th Annual Asian Conference and Exhibition on Geospatial Information, Technology and Applications (Singapore, August 2009)*.

Linkens, D. and Chen, M. (1999). Input selection and partition validation for fuzzy modelling using neural network. *Fuzzy Sets and Systems*, 107, 3 (1999), pp. 299–308.

Lomolino, M., Riddle, B., & Brown, J. (2009). *Biogeography*. Sinauer Associates.

Macfarlane, P. W. (2006) – Is electrocardiography still useful in the diagnosis of cardiac chamber hypertrophy and dilatation?, *Cardiology Clinics*, 24 (3), pp. 401-411, 2006

Magdic, K. S., Saul, L. M. (1997) – ECG Interpretation of chamber enlargement, *Critical Care Nurse*, 17 (1), 13, 16-25, 1997

Masson, J. M., Hancock, E. W., & Gettes, L. S. (2007) – AHA/ACC/HRS Scientific Statement, Recommendations for Standardization and Interpretation of the Electrocardiogram. Part II: Electrocardiography Diagnostic Statement List, A Scientific Statement From the American Heart Association Electrocardiography and Arrhythmias Committee, Council on Clinical Cardiology; The American College of Cardiology Foundation, and the Heart Rhythm Society, *Circulation*. 115: pp. 1325-1332, 2007

McKenna, W. J., Krikler, D. M., & Goodwin, J. F. (1982) – Arrhythmias in dilated and hypertrophic cardiomyopathy. *Medical Clinics of North America*, 68 (4), pp. 983-1000, 1984

Nauck, D., Klawonn, F., and Kruse, R. (1997). *Foundations of Neuro-Fuzzy Systems*. John Wiley & Sons.

Olson, E. N. (2004) – A decade of discoveries in cardiac biology, *Nature Medicine* 10, pp. 467-474, 2004

Ovreiu, M., Nair, B., Xu, M., Bakri, M., Li, L., Wazni, O., Fahmy, T., Petre, J., Sessler, D., Starr, N., & Bashour, A. (2008) Electrocardiographic Activity Before Onset of Postoperative Atrial Fibrillation in Cardiac Surgery Patients, *PACE*, November 2008, Vol. 31, issue 11, pp. 1371-1382 (with editorial comment of Lombardi, F. (2008) – "Atrial Fibrillation After cardiac Surgery: Prevention or Early Treatment of Patients at Risk", *PACE*, November 2008, Vol. 31, issue 11, pp. 1369-1370)

Panchal, V., Singh, P., Kaur, N., & Kundra, H. (2009). Biogeography based satellite image classification. *International Journal of Computer Science and Information Security*. 6, 2 (Nov. 2009), pp. 269–274.

Pereira, N., Barbosa, M., Ribeiro, A., Amorim, F., & Rocha, M. (2010) – Predictors of mortality in patients with dilated cardiomyopathy: Relevance of Chagas disease as an etiological factor, *Revista Espanola de Cardiologia*, 63 (7), pp. 788-797, 2010

Rahnamayan, S., Tizhoosh, H., & Salama, M. (2006). Opposition-based differential evolution for optimization of noisy problems, in *Proceedings of IEEE Congress on Evolutionary Computation (Vancounver, Canada, July 2006)*. pp. 1865–1872.

Rahnamayan, S., Tizhoosh, H., & Salama, M. (2007). Quasioppositional differential evolution, in *Proceedings of IEEE Congress on Evolutionary Computation (Singapore, September 2007)*. 2229–2236.

Rahnamayan, S., Tizhoosh, H., & Salama, M. (2008). Opposition-based differential evolution. *IEEE Transactions on Evolutionary Computation*, 12, 1 (2008), pp. 64–79.

Rarick, R., Simon, D., Villaseca, F. E., & Vyakaranam, B. (2009). Biogeography-based optimization and the solution of the power flow problem, In *Proceedings of the IEEE Conference on Systems, Man, and Cybernetics (San Antonio, Texas, October 2009)*. pp. 1029–1034.

Simon, D. (2002a). Training fuzzy systems with the extended Kalman filter. *Fuzzy Sets and Systems*, 132, 2 (December 2002), pp. 189–199.

Simon, D. (2002b). Training radial basis neural networks with the extended Kalman filter. *Neurocomputing*, 48, 1 (October 2002), pp. 455–475.

Simon, D. (2002c). Sum normal optimization of fuzzy membership functions. *International Journal of Uncertainty, Fuzziness, and Knowledge-Based Systems*, 10, 4 (August 2002), pp. 363–384.

Simon, D. (2005). H-infinity estimation for fuzzy membership function optimization, *International Journal of Approximate Reasoning*, 40, 3 (November 2005), pp. 224–242.

Simon, D. (2008). Biogeography-Based Optimization, *IEEE Transactions on Evolutionary Computation*, 12, 6 (December 2008), pp. 702–713.

Sox, H. C., Garber, A. M., & Littenberg, B. (1989). The resting Electrocardiogram as a Screening Test: A Clinical Analysis, *Annals of Internal Medicine*, 111, pp. 489-502, 1989

Tetko, I., Livingstone, D., & Luik, A. (1995). Neural network studies. 1. Comparison of overfitting and overtraining. *Journal of Chemical Information and Modeling*, 35, 5 (September 1995), pp. 826–833.

Tizhoosh, H. (2005). Opposition-based learning: A new scheme for machine intelligence, in *Proceedings of the International Conference on Computational Intelligence for Modelling, Control and Automation (Vienna, Austria, November 2005)*. pp. 695–701.

Visinescu, M., Bashour, A., Wazni, O., & Gopakumaran, B. (2004). Automatic detection of conducted premature atrial contractions to predict atrial fibrillation in patients after cardiac surgery, in *Proceedings of the 31st Annual International Conference on Computing in Cardiology (Chicago, Illinois, September 2004)*. pp. 429–432.

Visinescu, M. (2005). *Analysis of ECG to predict atrial fibrillation in post-operative cardiac surgical patients*. Doctoral dissertation, Cleveland State University, Cleveland, Ohio.

Visinescu, M., Bashour, A., Bakri, M., & Nair, B. (2006). Automatic detection of QRS complexes in ECG signals collected from patients after cardiac surgery, in *Proceedings of the 28th Annual International Conference of the IEEE Engineering in Medicine and Biology Society (New York, August 2006)*. pp. 3724–3727.

Ziegler, R. F. (1970). Electrocardiographic Clues in the diagnosis of congenital heart disease, *Cardiovascular Clinics*, 2 (1), pp. 97-114, 1970

Whittaker, R. (1998). *Island Biogeography*. Oxford University Press.

3

Prevention of Sudden Cardiac Death in Patients with Cardiomyopathy

M. Obadah Al Chekakie

University of Colorado, Cheyenne Regional Medical Center
United States

1. Introduction

Sudden cardiac death (SCD) is a major public health issue with an estimated annual incidence of 300,000 - 400,000 cases per year. The ACC/AHA/ESC 2006 guidelines define SCD as "death from an unexpected circulatory arrest, usually due to a cardiac arrhythmia occurring within an hour of the onset of symptoms"(Zipes et al. 2006). Most of the patients experiencing sudden cardiac arrest have an ejection fraction (LVEF) more than 50%, with the majority of these patients having a history of coronary artery disease (CAD). However, the risk of death in patients with LVEF of less than 35% is higher than patients with better preserved LVEF (Gorgels et al. 2003). Beta blocker therapy, Angiotensin enzymes inhibitors (ACE-I), angtiotensin receptor blockers as well as aldosteron antagonists have been shown to decrease the risk of sudden cardiac death especially in post myocardial infarction patients (Seidl et al. 1998; Domanski et al. 1999; Pitt et al. 2003; McMurray et al. 2005). In contrast antiarrhythmic drug therapy doesn't prevent sudden cardiac death in patients with cardiomyopathy. The focus of this chapter is to review the major implantable cardioverter defibrillator (ICD) and cardiac resynchronization therapy trials and their effects on sudden cardiac death prevention in patients with cardiomyopathy who are receiving optimal medical therapy.

2. Trials examining the benefits of ICD therapy in sudden cardiac death prevention

2.1 Secondary prevention trials of defibrillator therapy

The earlier trials examined the highest risk population of patients who had cardiac arrest due to ventricular fibrillation or sustained ventricular tachycardia (VT) and syncope. These trials helped establish the benefit of ICD therapy in prevention of sudden cardiac death as well as identify patients who are at high risk of dying suddenly and might benefit from ICD therapy as a primary prevention approach.

The first trial is the **Antiarrhythmic versus Implantable Defibrillators Trial (AVID)**. Patients were included if they were resuscitated from VT, had sustained VT with syncope or had sustained VT with LVEF < 40% and symptoms suggestive of hemodynamic compromise (angina or congestive heart failure or near syncope) (AVID 1997). Patients were excluded if the ventricular arrhythmia was due to a reversible cause, but those patients were followed in a registry. AVID enrolled 1016 patients and the primary end point was all cause mortality. Over

80% of the patients randomized to antiarrhythmic therapy (total of 509 patients) were on Amiodarone at end of follow up. AVID was terminated early when patients with ICD therapy (n=506) had a 38% reduction in all cause mortality compared to patients with antiarrhythmic drug therapy (HR 0.62, 95% CI of 0.47 to 0.81). Analysis of the AVID trial showed that patients with LVEF < 35% who received an ICD had significant reduction of sudden cardiac death while patients with LVEF > 35% who received an ICD did not see significant benefit compared to the antiarrhythmic drug therapy group (Domanski et al. 1999).

The patients with a reversible cause of ventricular arrhythmia who were not randomized were followed in a registry. These patients were in general younger, had a better mean LVEF and were more likely to have history of coronary artery disease and had underwent revascularization. Most of the reversible causes were due to ischemia or myocardial infarction (65%) or due to electrolytes imbalance (10%). Patients who were categorized as having VT/VF due to reversible causes had similar if not higher risk of sudden cardiac death compared to patients with no identifiable reversible cause(Wyse et al. 2001). Careful follow up and aggressive assessment for this patient group is advised.

The second study is the **Canadian Implantable Defibrillator Study (CIDS)**, which enrolled 659 patients who had VT, sustained VT with syncope or sustained VT with LVEF < 35%. Patients were excluded if they had recent myocardial infarction (MI) with in the past 72 hours or if they had electrolytes imbalance. Primary end point was all cause mortality. The patients were followed for an average of 36 months. There was a 20% relative risk reduction of death with ICD therapy compared to amiodarone (p=0.14)(Connolly et al. 2000). Analysis of CIDS showed that patients with low LVEF benefited from ICD therapy more than patient with better-preserved LVEF(O'Brien et al. 2001).

The third study is the **Cardiac Arrest Study Hamburg (CASH)**, which was a small trial randomizing 288 patients to ICD therapy with drug therapy. Inclusion criteria included patients successfully resuscitated from cardiac arrest due to documented sustained ventricular arrhythmia. Exclusion criteria included patients who had a cardiac arrest within 72 hours after MI or cardiac surgery or if they had a reversible cause due to electrolyte abnormality or proarrhythmic drug. There was a trend towards lower death with ICD therapy compared to drug therapy (23% relative risk reduction, p=0.16). Average follow up was 57 months. The lack of benefit in the CASH trial might be due to the fact that it had a small study population and better mean LVEF (45% ±18%) compared to the AVID trial(Kuck et al. 2000). Also, 44% of patient in CASH study had epicardial lead implantation as compared to only 4% in the AVID trial.

A pooled analysis of these trials demonstrated that all cause mortality was reduced by 27% (HR of ICD compared to Amiodarone of 0.73, 95% CI 0.60-0.87, p<0.001) (Connolly et al. 2000). Arrhythmic death was also reduced in the ICD group compared to the Amiodarone group (HR 0.49, 95% CI of 0.36 to 0.67, p<0.001). The metaanalysis also showed that patients with LVEF <35% had a significant benefit from ICD therapy compared to Amiodarone (HR 0.66, 95% CI of 0.53 to 0.83) while patients with LVEF >35% had no significant benefit from ICD therapy compared to Amiodarone therapy (HR of 1.2, 95% CI of 0.81 to 1.76). Furthermore, patients receiving epicardial lead systems had no benefit from ICD therapy compared to Amiodarone (HR 1.52, 95% CI of 0.92 to 2.50), while patients with transvenous lead had the most benefit (HR 0.69, 95% CI of 0.56 to 0.85). The three randomized trials examining the benefit of implantable cardioverter defibrillator (ICD) therapy in patients who survived cardiac arrest are summarized in Table 1.

Trial	N	Inclusion Criteria	Primary Endpoint	Age	Mean LVEF	HR (95% Confidence Interval)	P Value
Antiarrhythmics versus Implantable Defibrillators (AVID) (1016 patients)	1016	Resuscitated VF, sustained VT and syncope or sustained VT with LVEF < 40% and severe symptoms	All cause mortality	65	35%	0.62 (0.47-0.81)	0.02
Canadian Implatable Defibrillator Study (CIDS) (659 patients)	659	Resuscitated VF, sustained VT and syncope or sustained VT with LVEF < 35% or unmonitored syncope with subsequent inducible VT or sustained VT	All cause mortality	64	34%	0.82 (0.60 to 1.10)	0.14
Cardiac Arrest Study Hamburg (CASH)	288	cardiac arrest due to documented sustained ventricular arrhythmia	All cause mortality	58	45%		0.16

Table 1. Secondary prevention trials of ICD therapy. VT is for ventricular tachycardia, VF is for Ventricular Fibrillation, LVEF is for left Ventricular ejection Fraction. HR is for hazard Ratio, CI is confidence interval.

These trials established the benefits of ICD therapy in patients who survived cardiac arrest in the absence of reversible causes. Patients with reversible causes of the cardiac arrest remain high risk and should be followed closely. Even though the metaanalysis of these trials showed no benefits of ICD therapy in patients with LVEF >35%, this is not reflected in the guidelines due to the fact that LVEF was not an entry criterion in these trials. Furthermore, the mean time of cardiac arrest and measurement of LVEF was 3 days in the AVID trial, and the LVEF shortly after cardiac arrest might be depressed from myocardial injury and might improve over time. Table 2 lists current guidelines for ICD therapy.

Class I: (General agreement of benefit with ICD therapy)

1. ICD therapy is indicated in patients who are survivors of cardiac arrest due to VF or hemodynamically unstable sustained VT after evaluation to define the cause of the event and to exclude any completely reversible causes.
2. ICD therapy is indicated in patients with structural heart disease and spontaneous sustained VT, whether hemodynamically stable or unstable.
3. ICD therapy is indicated in patients with syncope of undetermined origin with clinically relevant, hemodynamically significant sustained VT or VF induced at electrophysiological study.
4. ICD therapy is indicated in patients with LVEF less than or equal to 35% due to prior

MI who are at least 40 days post-MI and are in NYHA functional Class II or III.

5. ICD therapy is indicated in patients with nonischemic dilated cardiomyopathy who have an LVEF less than or equal to 35% and who are in NYHA functional Class II or III.

6. ICD therapy is indicated in patients with LV dysfunction due to prior MI who are at least 40 days post-MI, have an LVEF less than or equal to 30%, and are in NYHA functional Class I.

7. ICD therapy is indicated in patients with nonsustained VT due to prior MI, LVEF less than or equal to 40%, and inducible VF or sustained VT at electrophysiological study.

Class IIa (Weight of evidence is in favor of usefulness of ICD therapy)

1. ICD implantation is reasonable for patients with unexplained syncope, significant LV dysfunction, and non-ischemic dilated cardiomyopathy.

2. ICD implantation is reasonable for patients with sustained VT and normal or near-normal ventricular function.

3. ICD implantation is reasonable for patients with hypertrophic cardiomyopathy (HCM) who have 1 or more major risk factors for SCD. [Major risk factors for SCD in patients with HCM are: prior cardiac arrest, spontaneous sustained VT, spontaneous non-sustained VT, Family history of SCD, LV thickness ≥ 30 mm and abnormal blood pressure response to exercise]

4. ICD implantation is reasonable for the prevention of SCD in patients with ARVD/C who have 1 or more risk factors for SCD. [Risk factors for SCD in patients with ARVD/C are: prior cardiac arrest, spontaneous sustained VT, spontaneous non-sustained VT, evidence of extensive RV disease, LV involvement, presentation with polymorphic VT and RV apical aneurysm and induction of VT during electrophysiologic testing]

5. ICD implantation is reasonable to reduce SCD in patients with long-QT syndrome who are experiencing syncope and/or VT while receiving beta blockers.

6. ICD implantation is reasonable for non hospitalized patients awaiting transplantation.

7. ICD implantation is reasonable for patients with Brugada syndrome who have had syncope.

8. ICD implantation is reasonable for patients with Brugada syndrome who have documented VT that has not resulted in cardiac arrest.

9. ICD implantation is reasonable for patients with catecholaminergic polymorphic VT who have syncope and/or documented sustained VT while receiving beta blockers.

10. ICD implantation is reasonable for patients with cardiac sarcoidosis, giant cell myocarditis, or Chagas disease.

Class IIb (Efficacy of the ICD therapy is less well established)

1. ICD therapy may be considered in patients with non-ischemic heart disease who have an LVEF of less than or equal to 35% and who are in NYHA functional Class I.

2. ICD therapy may be considered for patients with long-QT syndrome and risk factors for SCD.

3. ICD therapy may be considered in patients with syncope and advanced structural heart disease in whom thorough invasive and noninvasive investigations have failed

	to define a cause.
4.	ICD therapy may be considered in patients with a familial cardiomyopathy associated with sudden death.
5.	ICD therapy may be considered in patients with LV noncompaction.

Class III (General agreement that an ICD is not effective and may be harmful)

1. ICD therapy is not indicated for patients who do not have a reasonable expectation of survival with an acceptable functional status for at least 1 year, even if they meet ICD implantation criteria specified in the Class I, IIa, and IIb recommendations above.
2. ICD therapy is not indicated for patients with incessant VT or VF.
3. ICD therapy is not indicated in patients with significant psychiatric illnesses that may be aggravated by device implantation or that may preclude systematic follow-up.
4. ICD therapy is not indicated for NYHA Class IV patients with drug-refractory congestive heart failure who are not candidates for cardiac transplantation or CRT-D.
5. ICD therapy is not indicated for syncope of undetermined cause in a patient without inducible ventricular tachyarrhythmias and without structural heart disease.
6. ICD therapy is not indicated when VF or VT is amenable to surgical or catheter ablation (e.g., atrial arrhythmias associated with the Wolff-Parkinson-White syndrome, RV or LV outflow tract VT, idiopathic VT, or fascicular VT in the absence of structural heart disease).
7. ICD therapy is not indicated for patients with ventricular tachyarrhythmias due to a completely reversible disorder in the absence of structural heart disease (e.g., electrolyte imbalance, drugs, or trauma).

Table 2. Recommendations for ICD therapy based on the ACC/AHA/HRS 2008 Guidelines for Device Based Therapy.

2.2 Primary prevention trials of defibrillator therapy
2.2.1 Primary prevention of SCD in patients with ischemic cardiomyopathy with and without prior myocardial infarction

The earlier primary prevention trials used electrophysiologic testing as well as a reduced LVEF as part of entry criterion. Electrophysiologic testing (EP study) was thought to be a reliable method of risk stratification of patients with coronary artery disease (CAD) who survived myocardial infarction.

The First of these trials is the **First Multicenter Automatic Defibrillator Implantation Trial (MADIT- I)** which compared ICD therapy to conventional care in 196 patients post MI, LVEF < 35%, non-sustained VT on ambulatory monitoring and inducible VT by programmed electrical stimulation and failure of intravenous procainamide to prevent inducibility (Moss et al. 1996). Patients were excluded if they had prior cardiac arrest or syncope due to ventricular tachycardia (VT) not related to myocardial infarction (MI). Patients were also excluded if they had suffered myocardial infarction within 3 weeks of randomization, had coronary artery bypass surgery within 2 months of randomization or if they had angioplasty within 3 months of randomization. MADIT I started enrolling patients in December 1990, with only transthoracic implantation of ICD was available at the time. Nonthoracotomy transvenous leads were implanted after being approved in August of 1993. Of the 196 patients enrolled, 95 patients were assigned to the ICD group and 101 patients were assigned to the conventional medical therapy group (which also included use of antiarrhythmic drugs). Primary endpoint was all cause mortality. After a mean follow up of 27 months, patients assigned to the ICD group had lower mortality than patients assigned to the conventional treatment group (Hazard Ratio (HR) of 0.46, 95% confidence interval (CI) 0.26 to 0.82, p=0.009). The interval from last MI was > 6 months in 75% of patients in each treatment group. The benefit of ICD was similar in patients with thoracotomy and non-thoracotomy ICD implantation (p=0.78). MADIT-I trail was the first trail to include patients who had purely low LVEF and inducible non-suppressible sustained ventricular arrhythmias during electrophysiologic testing.

The First Multicenter Unsustained Tachycardia Trial (MUSTT-I) trial was designed to determine whether inducibilty of VT identified risk of sudden cardiac death in patients with LVEF < 40%, prior myocardial infarction and non-sustained VT documented more than 4 days after MI. Patients were enrolled if they had a positive electrophysiology study (defined as an inducible monomorphic VT or inducible polymorphic VT with one or two extrastimuli). Those with negative EP study were followed in a registry. A total of 704 patients with positive EP study were randomized to electrophysiologic guided antiarrhythmic therapy (which included a drug or implantation of an ICD) versus best medial therapy (mainly beta blockers and angiotensin enzyme inhibitors but no antiarrhythmic drug therapy) (Buxton et al. 1999). Patients who failed suppression of inducibility of the ventricular arrhythmia after at least one antiarrhythmic drug trial could receive an ICD. The ICD implantation was not randomized in MUSTT-I. The primary endpoint was cardiac arrest or death from arrhythmia. Secondary endpoints included death from all causes, death from cardiac causes and spontaneous sustained VT. Over a follow up period of 39 months, patients assigned to electrophysiologic testing (n=351) had lower risk of arrhythmic death or cardiac arrest compared to patients receiving best medical therapy (n=353) (Relative risk 0.73, 95% CI 0.53 to 0.99, p =0.04). This is mostly attributable to lower risk of arrhythmic death or cardiac arrest in patients receiving an ICD compared to patients not receiving an ICD (relative risk 0.24, 95% CI of 0.13 to 0.45, p< 0.001). Patients who received an ICD had a lower risk of all cause mortality compared to patients with electrophysiology guided therapy who received antiarrhythmic drugs only (Relative risk 0.42, 95% CI of 0.29 to 0.61) This remained significant even after adjusting for all other clinical variables (Figure 1).

MUSTT-I showed that patients who had an inducible VT that was suppressed with antiarrhythmic drugs did not have any mortality benefit.

Patients who were screened for MUSTT-I but had a negative EP study were followed in a registry. Data was available for 1397 patients after 39 months of follow up. Total mortality was compared in this registry with the 353 patients in MUSTT-I with positive EP study that were assigned to best medical therapy. Only 35% of patients in the registry were on beta blockers compared to 51% of patients with inducible arrhythmias assigned to no antiarrhythmic therapy. The rate of used of ACE-I was similar (72% and 77% respectively). At 39 months, mortality was higher in patients with positive EP study assigned to best medical therapy (48%) compared to the patients with negative EP study in the registry (44%), (unadjusted p=0.09, adjusted p<0.001 for other clinical factors including use of beta blockers). Even though this difference was statistically significant, the absolute difference of 4% over 5 years is not clinically meaningful. Given these results as well as the consistency of LVEF <35% to predict a mortality benefit from ICD therapy, Electrophysiologic testing is not routinely performed in patients with coronary artery disease and LVEF < 35% as a risk stratifying tool. (Buxton et al. 2000).

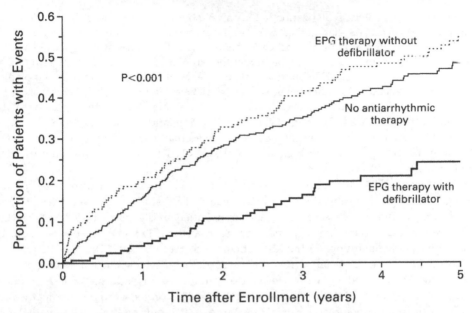

Fig. 1. Kaplan- Meier Estimates of the Rates of Death from All Causes. EPG denotes electrophysiologically guided. (From Buxton, A. E., Lee, K. L., Fisher, J. D., et al. (1999). "A randomized study of the prevention of sudden death in patients with coronary artery disease. Multicenter Unsustained Tachycardia Trial Investigators." New England Journal of Medicine, Vol. 341, No.25, (December, 1999): pp. 1882-1890, ISSN 0028-4793, with permission)

The Coronary Artery Bypass Graft Patch and The Second Multicenter Automatic Defibrillator Implantation Trial (MADIT- II) trials examined the benefits of ICD therapy in patients with reduced LVEF months after myocardial infarction and did not include electrophysiologic testing or arrhythmia suppression as part of entry criterion. **The Coronary Artery Bypass Graft-Patch Trial (CABG-Patch)** randomized 1055 patients undergoing coronary artery bypass surgery, LVEF <36% and positive signal-averaged electrocardiograms to receive ICD therapy (n=446) or conventional medical therapy (n=454) (Bigger 1997). Only 50% of the patients had prior myocardial infarction but all the patients received epicardial ICD systems. ICD therapy showed no survival benefit over conventional medical therapy (HR 1.06, 95% CI of 0.81 to 1.42, p=0.64). The lack of benefit of ICD therapy in this trial could be due to the methods used for patient selection, but most likely is due to the effects of complete revascularization on the risk of sudden cardiac death. In a subanalysis of **Studies of Left Ventricular Dysfunction (SOLVD)** trial, CABG was found to be associated with a 36% relative risk reduction of all cause mortality and a 46% reduction of sudden cardiac death regardless of the severity of heart failure or the decrease in the LVEF. This might have contributed to the lack of benefit from ICD early after coronary artery bypass surgery (Veenhuyzen et al. 2001).

The Second Multicenter Automatic Defibrillator Implantation Trial (MADIT- II) randomized 1232 patients in a 3:2 fashion with LVEF < 30% and prior MI to receive an ICD (n=742) compared to medical therapy (n=490). Patients were excluded if they had a recent MI

(<1 month), if they had revascularization in the past 3 months prior to randomization or if they were New York Heart Association (NYHA) class IV at enrollment. Mean follow up was for 30 months and primary end point was all cause mortality. ICD therapy was associated with a 31% reduction in relative risk of death at 20 months (HR 0.69, 95% confidence interval of 0.53 to 0.93, p = 0.02) (Moss et al. 2002). There was no difference in subgroup analysis based on age, gender, ejection fraction, QRS duration as well as NYHA class in terms of ICD benefit.

All ICD implantations were transvenous lead systems. No deaths were related to the implantation procedure and the complication of lead implantation was 1.8% and infection rate was 0.7%. Analysis of the mortality events showed that ICD therapy mainly prevented sudden cardiac death (HR 0.33, 95% CI of 0.2 to 0.53, p<0.001) but did not affect non-sudden cardiac death (p=0.32).

Even though MADIT-II did not require electrophysiologic testing as an entry criterion, the investigators sought to evaluate the predictive value of EP study to predict mortality and ICD efficacy as a pre-specified secondary endpoint. Patients assigned to the ICD group were encouraged to undergo an EP study and they received the ICD regardless of the results of the electrophysiologic testing. Of the 720 patients who received an ICD, only 593 patients underwent EP testing. A positive EP study was defined as sustained monomorphic or polymorphic VT induced with 3 or fewer extrastimuli or VF induced with 2 or fewer extrastimuli. A positive EP study according to this standard protocol did not predict the pre-specified primary endpoint of spontaneous VT or VF requiring treatment by the ICD (p=0.28). Patients with inducible VT were more likely to have VT during follow up (0.023) compared to patients with no inducible VT (Daubert et al. 2006). This confirms the findings of MUSTT-I trial in regards to the utility of EP testing in risk stratifying patients with coronary artery disease and LVEF < 35%.

Another subanalysis of MADIT-II trial showed that patients with ICD therapy who underwent coronary revascularization within 6 months of randomization had no survival benefit from ICD therapy compared to patients in the conventional treatment group (HR = 1.19; p = 0.76), while patients with ICD therapy who were randomized > 6 months after coronary revascularization had significant survival benefit from ICD therapy (HR =0.64, p = 0.01) after adjusting for other important clinical variables (Goldenberg et al. 2006). Furthermore, mortality risk in patients in MADIT II was shown to be time dependent, with benefit extending even for patients who had remote MI (>15 years) (Wilber et al. 2004). Two studies were conducted examine the benefits of ICD therapy early after myocardial infarction (MI). The first is **The Defibrillators in Acute Myocardial Infarction Trial (DINAMIT) which** was designed to evaluate the potential for ICD benefit early (6 to 40 days) after a MI in patients with LVEF <35%, and abnormal autonomic tone [high resting heart rate over 80 beats per minutes (bpm) or low heart rate variability]. Patients were excluded if they had three-vessel coronary intervention, if they already had an ICD or if they were planned to undergo coronary artery bypass graft surgery (CABG). A total of 647 patients were randomized to optimal medical therapy (n=342) or ICD therapy (n=332) (Hohnloser et al. 2004). The primary end point was all cause mortality and the secondary end point was arrhythmic death. After a mean follow up of 30 months, there was no overall survival benefit attributable to early implantation of an ICD compared to medical therapy [HR 1.08; 95% confidence interval (CI), 0.76 to 1.55; P=0.66]. The ICD group had less arrhythmic death compared to the medical therapy group (HR in the ICD group, 0.42; 95% CI, 0.22 to 0.83; P=0.009). There was an increase in non-sudden cardiac death in the ICD group compared to the medical therapy group (HR = 1.75; 95% CI, 1.11 to 2.76; P=0.02).

The second trial is **the Immediate Risk Stratification Improves Survival (IRIS) Trial**, which was a randomized, open label multicenter trial that studied the benefit of ICD therapy early after MI compared to optimal medical therapy. Patients were included if they had a history of myocardial infarction (5 to 31 days after MI), LVEF < 40% with either a baseline heart rate of > 90 bpm, non-sustained VT at >150 bpm on holter or both. A total of 898 patients were enrolled in the trial. Mean follow up was for 37 months, and almost 75% of the patients underwent revascularization. Most of the patients were on beta blockers (97% in the ICD group and 95% in the control group) and angiotensin receptor blockers (90% in ICD group and 91.1% in the control group). There was no difference in overall mortality between ICD group and the medical treatment group (HR 1.04, 95% CI of 0.81 to 1.35, p=0.78) (Steinbeck et al. 2009). Patients assigned to ICD therapy had lower incidence of sudden cardiac death (HR 0.55, 95% CI of 0.31 to 1.00, p = 0049) but higher incidence of non-sudden cardiac death (HR 1.92, 95% CI of 1.29 to 2.84).

The reasons for the lack of benefit of ICD therapy early after MI might never be known. Revascularization has a protective effect and leads to reverse remodeling especially if done in a timely fashion early after MI. Patients who died early in DINAMIT had pump failure. Other possibilities include side effects for ICD implantation early after MI or the negative effects of shocks or antitachycardia pacing on myocardial contractility.

In summary, the above trials support the use of ICD therapy for primary prevention of SCD in chronic ischemic cardiomyopathy. For patients who suffered a recent MI (<40 days), both IRIS and DINAMIT showed a decrease in arrhythmic death but no difference in all cause mortality. Currently, the guidelines support ICD therapy in patients with CAD who are > 40 days post MI and have LVEF < 35%.

Table 3 summarized the primary prevention trials in patients with coronary artery disease.

2.2.2 Primary prevention of SCD in patients with non-ischemic cardiomyopathy

The early trials examining the effects of ICD therapy compared to antiarrhythmic therapy in patients with non-ischemic cardiomyopathy (NICM) were small and not powered enough to show mortality benefit. The first trial is the **Amiodarone versus Implantable Cardioverter Defibrillator Trial (AMIOVERT)** which compared ICD therapy in 103 patients with NICM (with the diagnosis made > 6 months before enrollment) and non-sustained VT to amiodarone. The primary endpoint was all cause mortality. There was no difference in survival between the ICD group and the amiodarone group. The trial was terminated due to futility. The second trial is the **The Cardiomyopathy trial (CAT)** which was carried out in Germany and enrolled 104 patients with non-ischemic cardiomyopathy who were diagnosed within 9 months of enrollment. Mean follow up was 5.5 years and the primary end point was all cause mortality. Again there was no difference in survival between the ICD group and the control group. Both AMIOVERT and CAT trials were underpowered to detect a difference between groups, and in both of them the observed mortality was far lower than the predicted mortality used to design these trials.

Trial	N	Inclusion Criteria	Primary Endpoint	Age	Mean LVEF	NYHA Class	HR (95% CI)	P Value
First Multicenter Automatic Defibrillator Implantation Trial (MADIT-I)	196	NYHA I-III HF LVEF<35% MI > 4 weeks CABG > 3 months spontaneous NSVT and inducible VT	All cause mortality	63	26%	I, II and III	0.46 (0.26 to 0.82)	0.009
Multicenter Unsustained Tachycardia Trial (MUSTT)	704	NYHA I-III LVEF <40% MI>4 days spontaneous NSVT and inducible VT	Cardiac arrest or death from arrhythmia	65	28%	I, II and III	0.73 (0.53 -0.99)	0.04
The Coronary Artery Bypass Graft-Patch Trial (CABG-Patch)	1055	LVEF < 36%, Abnormal SAECG, undergoing CABG	All cause mortality	64	27%		1.06 (0.81 to 1.42)	0.64
Second Multicenter Automatic Defibrillator Implantation Trial (MADIT-II)	1232	NYHA I-III, LVEF < 30% MI > 1 month	All Cause mortality	64	23%	I, II and III	0.69 (0.53 to 0.93)	0.02
Defibrillators in Acute Myocardial Infarction Trial (DINAMIT)	674	NYHA I-III LVEF <35% recent MI (6-40 days) with depressed heart rate variability or elevated average Hear rate over 24 hrs	All Cause mortality	62	28%	I, II and III	1.08 (0.76 to 1.55)	0.66
the Immediate Risk Stratification Improves Survival (IRIS)	898	NYHA I-III LVEF <40% Recent MI (5 to 31 days after MI), with either a baseline heart rate of > 90 (bpm) or NSVT at >150 bpm on holter or both	All Cause mortality	62	30%	I, II and III	1.04 (0.81 to 1.35)	0.78

Table 3. Primary prevention trials of ICD therapy in patients with coronary artery disease. VT is for ventricular tachycardia, VF is for Ventricular Fibrillation, NSVT is for non sustained VT, LVEF is for left Ventricular ejection Fraction. HR is for hazard Ratio, CI is confidence interval.

The Defibrillators in Non-Ischemic Cardiomyopathy Treatment Evaluation Trial (DEFINITE) studied the efficacy of ICD therapy to prevent all cause mortality in patients with LVEF < 35% and non-sustained VT or frequent premature ventricular contractions (PVCs) on ambulatory monitoring (Kadish et al. 2004). A total of 488 patients (229 in the ICD group and 229 in the conventional treatment group) were enrolled and the primary end point was death from any cause and the secondary endpoint was sudden cardiac death. Most of the patients were receiving beta blocker (85%) and ACE-I (86%) There was a 35% relative risk reduction in mortality in the ICD group compared to the medical therapy group (HR, 0.65; 95% CI, 0.40 to

1.06; P=0.08) but it did not reach statistical significance. A significant reduction in SCD was observed (HR 0.20; 95% CI, 0.06 to 0.71; P=0.006). The DEFINITE trial didn't specify duration of heart failure as an entry criterion and it only required absence of a reversible cause of cardiomyopathy for enrollment. Patients in DEFINITE who had a recent diagnosis of non-ischemic cardiomyopathy (Using a 3 months cut point or a 9 months cut point) had similar benefit from ICD therapy when compared to patients who had a remote diagnosis of non-ischemic cardiomyopathy (p0.25) (Kadish et al. 2006)

The largest trial conducted to examine the effects of ICD therapy on sudden cardiac death prevention in patients with ischemic and non-ischemic cardiomyopathy is the **Sudden Cardiac Death-Heart Failure (SCD-HeFT) trial**. This trial enrolled 2521 patients with LVEF < 35%, NYHA II-III and it had similar proportion of patients with ischemic cardiomyopathy (52%) and non-ischemic cardiomyopathy (48%). Patients were randomized to receive a single chamber ICD (n=829), Amiodarone (n=845) or placebo (n=847) (Bardy et al. 2005). Patients with recent MI or revascularization (<1 month) were not eligible. Nearly 96% of patients were on ACE-I or angiotensin receptor blockers and 69% were receiving beta-blocker therapy. The primary endpoint was all cause mortality. The ICD group was programmed to shock therapy only. After mean follow up of 45.5 months, the ICD group had lower mortality compared to placebo (HR 0.77, 95% CI of 0.62-0.96, p=0.007) while amiodarone had no effect on mortality compared to placebo (HR 1.06, 95% CI 0.86 to 1.30, p=0.53) (Figure 2). Annual rate of appropriate ICD shocks occurred in 68% of patients with an average annual rate of 5.1%. The absolute reduction in mortality was similar in patients with ischemic (7.2%) and non-ischemic cardiomyopathy (6.5%).

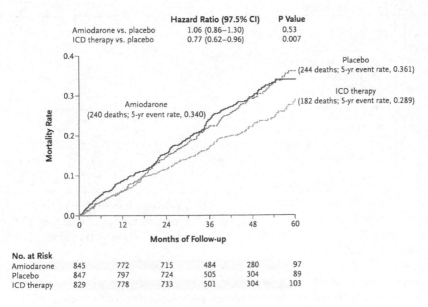

Fig. 2. Kaplan-Meier Estimates of Death from Any Cause. CI denotes confidence interval. (From Bardy, G. H., Lee, K. L., Mark, D. B., et al. (2005). "Amiodarone or an implantable cardioverter-defibrillator for congestive heart failure." New England Journal of Medicine Vol. 352, No.3, (January, 2005): pp. 225-237, ISSN 1533-4406, with permission).

In a pooled analysis of 10 primary prevention trials (AMIOVERT, MADIT-I, MUSTT, MADIT-II, CABG PATCH, CAT, SCD-HeFT, COMPANION, DEFINITE and DINAMIT), ICD therapy was associated with 25% relative risk reduction of all cause mortality (RRR 9% to 37%, p=0.003) compared to the medical treatment group. The absolute risk reduction was 7.9%, which means 13 ICDs need to be implanted to save one life over about 3 years. This was not sensitive to removal of the any of the trials from the analysis. The benefit of ICD therapy in sudden cardiac death prevention is above and beyond the mortality benefit associated with use of beta blocker and ACE-I in patients with systolic heart failure (Nanthakumar et al. 2004). Table 4 summarized the primary prevention trials of ICD therapy in patients with non-ischemic cardiomyopathy.

Trial (N)	N	Inclusion Criteria	Primary Endpoint	Age	Mean LVEF	NYHA Class	HR (95% CI)	P Value
Amiodarone Versus Implantable Cardioverter Defibrillator Trial (AMIOVERT)	103	NYHA I-IV LVEF < 35% Dilated cardiomyopathy, NSVT	All cause mortality	52	23%	I, II ,III and IV		0.80
Cardiomyopathy Trial (CAT)	104	NYHA II-III, LVEF < 30%, Dilated cardiomyopathy, Recent onset heart failure < 9 months	All cause mortality	52	24%	II and III		0.54
The Defibrillators in Non-Ischemic Cardiomyopathy Treatment Evaluation Trial (DEFINITE)	488	NYHA I-III, LVEF < 35%, Dilated cardioyopathy, NSVT or frequent PVCs (>10 PVC /hr)	All cause mortality	58	21%	I, II and III	0.65 (0.40 to 1.06)	0.08
Sudden Cardiac Death-Heart Failure (SCD-HeFT) trial	2521	NYHA II-III, EF< 35%, non-recent MI or revascularization (>1 month), non-recent heart failure onset (> 3 months)	All Cause mortality	60	25%	II and III	0.77 (0.62-0.96)	0.007

Table 4. Primary prevention trials of ICD therapy in patients with non-ischemic cardiomyopathy. VT is for ventricular tachycardia, VF is for Ventricular Fibrillation, PVC is for premature ventricular contractions, LVEF is for left Ventricular ejection Fraction. HR is for hazard Ratio, CI is confidence interval.

2.2.3 Cost effectiveness of ICD therapy

ICD therapy adds to the costs of care of patients with cardiomyopathy. Analysis of cost effectiveness in the SCD-HeFT trial showed that ICD therapy is cost effective, with incremental cost of $38,400 (95% CI of $25,217 to $80,160). This was similar in patients with ischemic and non-ischemic cardiomyopathy (Mark et al. 2006). In a pooled analysis of eight primary prevention trials, ICD therapy was not found to be cost effective in CABG PATCH and in DINAMIT, which are the trials that showed no mortality benefit from ICD therapy compared to conventional medical therapy. When examining the primary prevention trials that showed mortality benefit (MADIT-I, MUSTT, MADIT-II, COMPANION, DEFINITE and SCD-HeFT), ICD therapy was found to be cost effective, adding between 1.01 and 2.99 quality-adjusted life years with costs ranging from $34,000 to $70,200. This analysis takes into account that the ICD generator will be replaced every 5 years and assumes that the mortality benefit persists throughout the patient's life time (Sanders et al. 2005). Careful patient selection with a focus on patients who best fit the trials and are likely to die from arrhythmia and not from other non cardiac causes is important to insure the best utilization of this important and life saving therapy.

3. Defibrillator therapy in less common types of cardiomyopathy

Some of the inherited cardiomyopathies carry an increased risk of sudden cardiac death. We will review in this section the data behind ICD therapy in patients with two inherited disorders, first is Hypertrophic cardiomyopathy (HCM) and the second is arrhythmogenic right ventricular dysplasia./ cardiomyopathy (ARVD/C).

3.1 Hypertrophic cardiomyopathy
Hypertrophic cardiomyopathy is an autosomal dominant disorder diagnosed by two-dimensional echocardiography and is characterized by hypertrophied and non-dilated LV in the absence of other causes of hypertrophy (no history of hypertension or aortic stenosis or any other cardiac or systemic disease causing hypertrophy) (Maron 2002; 2003). Histologically, there is myocardial disarray, abnormal microvascular circulation with mismatch between myocardial mass and blood supply as well as interstitial fibrosis (Maron et al. 1986; Varnava et al. 2001). All of these predispose to ventricular tachycardia and ventricular fibrillation putting the patients at risk of sudden cardiac death (Varnava et al. 2001). The disease can present at any age in life. Earlier registries from tertiary care centers overestimated the risk of sudden cardiac death due to selection bias (with the annual risk of death thought to be 3 to 6%). More recent population studies of unselected patients from community centers suggest a more benign prognosis (annual risk of death of 1%) (Maron et al. 1999; Kofflard et al. 2003). Despite all recent data, there is a subset of patients with HCM who are at high risk of sudden cardiac death. In fact HCM remains the most common etiology for SCD in patients younger than 40 years and it can be the first presentation in patients with HCM (Maron 2003). Patients who survived a cardiac arrest are particularly at high risk of dying suddenly. Data from registries suggest a number of markers that increase the risk of sudden cardiac death. These markers include one or more of the following: LV wall thickness > 30 mm (Maron et al. 1999), syncope (particularly exertional syncope) (Kofflard et al. 2003), family history of SCD, non-sustained VT on ambulatory holter of > 120 bpm and a blunted blood pressure response to exercise. High LV outflow gradient (> 30 mmHg) has also been considered as risk marker for sudden cardiac death (Maron et al. 2003).
There are no randomized trials examining the benefits of ICD therapy in this patient population, so the data supporting ICD therapy is derived from registry data in patients with HCM who received an ICD when found to be high risk by their treating cardiologist / Electrophysiologist (Maron et al. 2000). The last update from the registry included 506 patients with HCM with a mean age of 42 years. Patients received and ICD if they had

survived a cardiac arrest due to ventricular tachycardia or ventricular fibrillation (secondary prevention cohort of 123 patients) or if they had one or more risk factors of sudden cardiac death: unexplained syncope, family history of sudden cardiac death in one or more first degree relatives, massive LV hypertrophy or non-sustained VT on holter monitoring (Primary prevention cohort of 383 patients) (Maron et al. 2007). Based on this registry, patients with HCM who survived cardiac arrest have a high appropriate ICD discharges (10.6% per year). This risk is lower in patients with HCM who had an ICD for primary prevention (3.6% per year). A third of these patients were 30 years or younger. Amiodarone was used based on the physicians judgment and it did not prevent arrhythmia occurrence (27% of patients who were on amiodarone had appropriate shocks). A third of the patients who received an ICD for primary prevention and had appropriate ICD discharges had one risk factor only for sudden cardiac death. There was no difference between the risk factors in the prediction of SCD. Since this is a young population of patients, they are at risk of inappropriate shocks, which occurred in 27% of the patients and were mainly due to sinus tachycardia, atrial fibrillation or lead malfunction. ICD implantation was shown to be safe with a rate of infection of 3.8% and the rate of lead fracture or dislodgement of 6.7%. Implantation of ICD has become an acceptable therapy in patients with HCM who survived cardiac arrest or who have two or more of the aforementioned risk factors of sudden cardiac death. For patients with only one risk factor of sudden cardiac death, the decision to implant an ICD is left to the physician's judgment and a careful discussion with the patient and his / her family in regards to the risks, benefits and alternatives of ICD therapy. In our experience, the presence of only one risk factor for SCD does not guarantee a recommendation for implanting an ICD. The clinical scenario is to be taken into account, as well as the patient's age and his / her wishes. The decision to implant is more favorable in a young patient with HCM with family history of sudden cardiac death or in a young patient with severe LV wall thickness (>30 mm) but still the discussion should take into account the young age of the patient and his / her wishes. On the other hand the discussion is more careful in an old patient with HCM in his / her 60s with history of non-exertional syncope that seems to be vasovagal in origin, the fact that the patient survived to that age without any major cardiac arrest indicates a more benign prognosis. Table 2 lists the current recommendations for ICD implantation for patients with hypertrophic cardiomyopathy.

3.2 Arrhythmogenic Right Ventricular Dysplasia / Cardiomyopathy (ARVD/C)

Arrhythmogenic right ventricular Dysplasia/ Cardiomyopathy (ARVD/C) is an inherited myopathy characterized by fibrofatty infiltration of the right ventricular (RV) wall, with left ventricular involvement over time in some patients (Gemayel et al. 2001; Sen-Chowdhry et al. 2004). The RV wall becomes thin, and the most areas affected are the RV inflow, apex and RV outflow, which form what is called the triangle of dysplasia. Ventricular tachycardia in general has left bundle branch morphology and is caused by macro-reentry and there is evidence that adrenergic stimulation acts as a trigger for these arrhythmias (Leclercq et al. 1996). ARVC/D accounts for 3 to 10% of death occurring in patients younger than 65 years (Tabib et al. 2003) and is one of the causes of sudden cardiac death in athletes (Maron 2003). The Most common presentation is with palpitations (due to frequent ventricular ectopy and ventricular tachycardia), chest pain, and syncope (mostly exertional). With time patients might develop RV dilatation, LV involvement and heart failure. Most of the data are obtained from registries in the United States and Europe (either single centers or multicenter registries). Diagnosis of

ARVD/C is based on the European Task Force criteria (McKenna et al. 1994). Risk factors of sudden cardiac death include prior cardiac arrest, hemodyamically unstable VT and prior syncope. Some studies suggested that LV involvement, development of heart failure and marked RV dilatation are risk factors for sudden cardiac death (Hulot et al. 2004). The role of electrophysiologic testing in risk stratification is less clear, with some studies showing a high positive predictive value and some showing low positive and low negative predictive values in predicting arrhythmias and appropriate ICD shocks (Corrado et al. 2003; Roguin et al. 2004). Beta blockers and sotalol were thought to be the best in suppressing these arrhythmias; however, this is challenged in more recent studies (Marcus et al. 2009). ICD therapy is clearly indicated in patients who survived cardiac arrest or have sustained VT and is a class IIa indication in patients with ARVD/C who have unexplained syncope. Some patients experience repetitive shocks requiring administration of antiarrhythmic drug therapy as well as VT ablation. Since this is a young population, they are also likely to experience inappropriate shocks due to sinus tachycardia or other supraventricular arrhythmias. In general ICD therapy is life saving and is well tolerated and has become accepted standard of care in patients with ARVD/C who experience cardiac arrest, sustained VT, unexplained syncope or marked RV dilatation or LV involvement (Epstein et al. 2008). Table 2 lists the current guidelines for ICD implantation in this patient population.

4. Cardiac Resynchronization Therapy (CRT) in patients with heart failure and its effects on mortality

Cardiac Resynchronization Therapy (CRT) aims at correcting mostly intraventricular dyssynchrony by stimulating the left ventricle (preferably basal stimulation) or by simultaneously stimulating the left and right ventricles after a sensed or paced atrial beat or during atrial fibrillation. CRT has been shown to improve the cardiac hemodynamics in patients with systolic heart failure, including improvements in the systolic blood pressure and decrease in the pulmonary capillary wedge pressure (by up to 20% in some patients) (Blanc et al. 1997). The early trials had endpoints related to heart failure functional status (including the 6 minute walk test, NYHA functional class), LV systolic function and improvement in the LV dimensions (including LVEF, LV end systolic volume and LV end systolic volume index as well as LV end diastolic dimension). Other studies relied on clinical composite score (which combines death from any cause, recent hospitalization for heart failure, NYHA class as well as the global assessment score) to define response to CRT (Chung et al. 2008). However, there is poor correlation between clinical and echocardiographic measurements of response and there is disagreement about the best way to measure response in patients with heart failure receiving CRT (Fornwalt et al.). So far QRS duration remains an important criterion for patient selection for CRT. Kass and colleagues demonstrated that baseline QRS duration correlated with enhancement in the isovolumetric dP/dt_{max} ($r = 0.6$, $p = 0.02$), while changes in the QRS duration with pacing did not predict hemodynamic response (Nelson et al. 2000). Most of the trials on CRT involved patients with systolic heart failure with LVEF < 35% and NYHA class III or IV as well as a QRS duration of > 120 msec. A trial studying patients with narrow QRS in patients with systolic heart failure failed to show any benefit. Later studies included patients with NYHA class I and class II heart failure with endpoints related to death or hospitalization. This section will focus mainly on the studies that included mortality as an endpoint.

4.1 Cardiac resynchronization therapy trials in patients with moderate to severe heart failure

The Multicenter InSync Randomized Clinical Evaluation (MIRACLE) trial involved implanting a CRT only device (with biventricular pacing only, no Defibrillator component). Patients were randomized if they had an LVEF < 35% and NYHA functional class III or IV heart failure despite optimal medical therapy and QRS duration of > 130 milliseconds (msec). a total of 453 patients were randomized after successful implantation of a CRT device to CRT ON (228 patients) and CRT OFF (225 patients) status for a period of 6 months (Abraham et al. 2002). The primary endpoint included the 6 minute walk test, quality of life score and NYHA class. A total of 453 patients were enrolled in the study. Patients assigned to CRT ON had 13% improvement in the 6-minute walk and in the quality of life score. The secondary endpoints also improved in the CRT ON arm including improvement in LVEF as well as peak oxygen consumption (VO2). The protocol specified safety variables that included an analysis of death or worsening heart failure. There was no difference in overall mortality (HR 0.73, 95% CI 0.34 to 1.54, p=0.40) but there was a decrease in hospitalization (HR 0.50, 95% CI 0.28 to 0.88, p= 0.02). The study did not specify mortality as a primary end point and was not powered enough to show differences in mortality.

The Multicenter Insync ICD randomized Clinical Evaluation (MIRACLE ICD) trial had a similar design to the MIRACLE study. Patients were included if they had LVEF < 35%, NYHA class III to IV despite optimal medical therapy and QRS duration of > 130 milliseconds and were at high risk of death from ventricular arrhythmias (Young et al. 2003). Almost two thirds of patients had an ischemic etiology and at least 60% were on beta blockers. All patients received a CRT-D device (total of 369 patients) of whom 182 had CRT OFF (controls) and 187 had CRT ON. At 6 months follow up, all patients with the CRT ON showed an improvement in the NYHA class (p=0.007) and the quality of life score (p=0.02). There was no difference in 6-minute walk distance (p=0.36) compared to the control group. Of the secondary endpoints, There was an improvement in the peak VO2 (p=0.04) and a trend towards reductions in the LV end systolic and end diastolic dimensions (p=0.06 for both) compared to the control group. The study did not show any difference in mortality (p=0.96) or hospitalization (p=0.69) between the two groups. Similar the to MIRACLE study, the MIRACLE ICD study had short follow up and was not powered enough to detect difference in mortality.

The CONTACT CD Biventricular Pacing study enrolled 490 patients with LVEF <35%, QRS > 120 msec and NYHA class II to IV despite optimal medical therapy and conventional indications for ICD implantation. Patients were assigned to CRT ON (245 patients) and CRT OFF (245 patients) for up to 6 months (Higgins et al. 2003). The primary endpoint was progression of heart failure, defined as all cause mortality, hospitalization for HF and ventricular tachycardia or ventricular fibrillation requiring device intervention. Secondary endpoints included peak oxygen consumption (VO2), 6-minute walk, NYHA class, quality of life as well as echocardiographic analysis. Patients with CRT ON had a 15% reduction in the composite HF progression but this was not statistically significant (p=0.35). However, patients with NYHA class III and IV had an improvement in the peak VO2 (p=0.003), 6-minute walk (p=0.03), NYHA class (p=0.0006) and QOL (0.02). Patients who had NYHA class I or II didn't show any improvement in any of the secondary parameters. One important finding in CONTACT CD trial is that patients with CRT ON had significant reductions in LV internal diameter in diastole (LVIDd) (p<0.001) LV internal diameter in systole (LVIDs) (p<0.001), and LVEF (p=0.02). Even patients with NYHA II had significant improvement in the LV dimensions with CRT ON. The study was not adequately powered to detect a statistical difference in the primary endpoint of composite HF progression. This was due to the fact that the observed event rates were half the expected while designing the trial.

The Comparison of Medical Therapy, Pacing and Defibrillation on Heart Failure Study (COMPANION) enrolled 1520 patients with LVEF< 35%, NYHA class III or IV heart failure despite optimal medical therapy and QRS duration of > 120 msec in a 1:2:2 fashion to medical therapy versus biventricular pacing alone (CRT only) versus biventricular pacing with defibrillation (CRT-D) (Bristow et al. 2004). Almost 59% of the patients had ischemic cardiomyopathy and 82% were NYHA class III. The primary endpoint was death or hospitalization for any cause while the secondary endpoints included death from any cause. As compared to the medical therapy group, patients with CRT only (Biventricular pacemaker only) decreased the risk of death or hospitalization from any cause (HR 0.81, p=0.014) as did CRT-D group (biventricular defibrillator group) (HR 0.80, p-0.01). CRT only decreased the risk of death by 24% (p=0.059) while CRT-D decreased the risk of death by 36% (p=0.003). COMPANION was the first trial to show that CRT improves the quality of life, symptoms as well as decrease the risk of death or hospitalization for heart failure.

The Cardiac Resynchronization-Heart Failure Study (CARE HF) randomized 813 patients with LVEF < 35%, NYHA class III to IV heart failure despite optimal medical therapy and QRS duration > 120 msec (patients with QRS between 120 to 149 msec had to have two of the three echocardiographic parameters of dys-synchrony: an aortic pre-ejection delay of > 140 msec, an interventricular mechanical delay of > 40 msec or delayed activation of the posterolateral wall of the LV (Cleland et al. 2005). Patients assigned to the CRT group received biventricular pacemaker (no defibrillators). The primary endpoint was the composite of death or unplanned hospitalization for a major cardiovascular event. Secondary endpoint was death from any cause. Other secondary endpoints included quality of life, improvement in NYHA class and echocardiographic parameters (mainly ventricular function, mitral regurgitation). After a mean follow up of 29.4 months, patients treated with CRT (total of 409 patients) had less death or hospitalization for cardiovascular event (HR 0.63, 95% CI 0.51 to 0.77, p< 0.001) compared to patients with medical therapy only (404 patients). CRT also improved survival (HR 0.64, 95% CI 0.48 to 0.85, p< 0.002) (Figure 3). Patients with CRT had improvement in NYHA class, better QOL, and showed smaller area of mitral regurgitation and an improvement in the LVEF at 3 and 18 months post CRT. CARE HF was the first CRT only trial to show that biventricular pacing alone can improve survival. The lack of mortality benefit from CRT only arm in COMPANION might be due to the fact that patients in COMPANION trial were sicker, with over 55% having ischemic cardiomyopathy with mean LVEF of 22% while patients in CARE HF had a mean LVEF of 25% and only a third of them had ischemic cardiomyopathy. The added benefits of CRT on survival will be examined later by the RAFT study.

The Cardiac Resynchronization Therapy in Patients with Heart Failure and Narrow QRS (RethinQ) study randomized 172 patients with history of NYHA class III heart failure, LVEF <35% despite optimal medical therapy and QRS duration of <130 msec with evidence of mechanical dys-synchrony on echocardiography (defined as septal to lateral or septal to inferior wall delay >65 msec as measured by tissue doppler or septal to posterior wall delay >130 msec as measured by M Mode echocardiography (Beshai et al. 2007). Primary outcome was the improvement of peak oxygen consumption of > 1 ml per kilogram of body weight

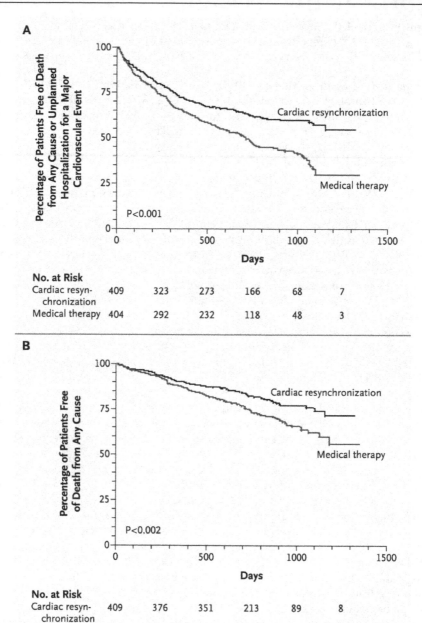

Fig. 3. Kaplan-Meier Estimates of the Time to the Primary End point of death or unplanned hospitalization for a major cardiovascular event (Panel A) and Death from any cause (Panel B). *(From Cleland, J. G., Daubert, J. C., Erdmann, E., et al. (2005). "The effect of cardiac resynchronization on morbidity and mortality in heart failure." New England Journal of Medicine, Vol. 352, No.15, (April, 2005): pp. 1539-1549, ISSN 1533-4406, with permission).*

per minute during cardiopulmonary exercise testing. The secondary outcomes were improvements in the 6 minute walk test, NYHA class and quality of life. All patients had a CRT device implantation and were assigned to CRT ON (n=76) or no CRT (n=80). After follow up of 6 months, there was no difference in the primary endpoint between patients with CRT and patients with no CRT (46% vs 44%, p=0.63). Patients in the CRT group with a QRS > 120 msec had significant improved in peak oxygen consumption at 6 months follow up (0.02) but patients in the CRT group with QRS <120 msec didn't have improvement in peak oxygen consumption at 6 months (p=0.45). There was no improvement in the quality of life measures (as measured by Minnesota living with Heart failure questionnaire) and in the 6-minute walk test in both groups of patients regardless of the QRS duration. Patients with CRT on had an improvement in the NYHA class at 6 months compared to patients with no CRT regardless of the QRS duration (p=0.006).

4.2 Cardiac resynchronization therapy trials in patients with mild heart failure

The Resynchronization Reverses Remodeling in Systolic Left Ventricular Dysfunction Study (REVERSE) trial was the first CRT trial to include patients with NYHA II and asymptomatic NYHA class I patients with LV dysfunction. A total of 610 patients underwent CRT device implantation and were randomized to CRT ON (419 patients) and CRT OFF (191 patients). Inclusion criteria included LVEF <40%, NYHA functional class I or II heart failure with a QRS 120 msec (Linde et al. 2008). Mean follow up was for 12 months. The primary end point was the heart failure (HF) clinical composite response (which included heart failure hospitalization, NYHA class and global assessment score). Secondary endpoints included LV end-systolic volume index and hospitalization for worsening HF. There was no difference between the two groups in the HF clinical composite score (which compared only the percent worsened) (p = 0.10). Patients assigned to CRT-ON experienced a greater improvement in LV end-systolic volume index (–18.4 ± 29.5 ml/m² vs. –1.3 ± 23.4 ml/m², p < 0.0001) and had a 53% relative risk reduction in time to first HF hospitalization (p=0.03). There was no difference between the two groups in the 6- minute walk test and in the quality of life scores. The improvement in LV end systolic volume index was similar in patients with NYHA I and NYHA II. The rate of LV lead implantation related complications was 10%. These complications were mostly due to LV lead dislodgement or diaphragmatic stimulation.

The Multicenter Automatic Defibrillator Implantation Trial with Cardiac Resynchronization therapy (MADIT-CRT) randomized 1820 patients with LVEF <30%, NYHA class I or II HF and QRS duration of > 130 msec in a 3:2 design to cardiac resynchronization therapy with defibrillation capacity (CRT-D) (1089 patients) and to ICD only group (731 patients). The primary endpoint was death from any cause or hospitalization for heart failure (Moss et al. 2009). Secondary endpoints included death from any cause and heart failure hospitalization alone. Follow up was for 4.5 years. Patients who received CRT-D had lower risk of death or hospitalization for heart failure (HR 0.66, 95% CI of 0.52 to 0.84, p=0.001) compared to the ICD only group. There was no difference in death from any cause between the two groups (HR 1.00, 95% CI of 0.69-1.44, p=0.99). The rate of hospitalization was significantly lower in the CRT-D group compared to the ICD only group (HR 0.59, 95% CI of 0.47 to 0.74, p<0.001). Patients with ischemic and non-ischemic cardiomyopathy benefited similarly from CRT. Subanalysis of MADIT CRT showed that female patients (n=453, 25%) were more likely to have non-ischemic cardiomyopathy and left bundle branch block (LBBB) compared to male patients. Female patients were more likely to have reverse remodeling by echocardiography and had a 69% relative risk reduction of death or heart failure (HR of 0.31, p<0.001) (Arshad et al.). Patients with QRS duration > 150 msec had greater benefit from CRT (HR 0.48, 95% CI 0.37 to 0.64) compared to patients with QRS duration < 150 msec (HR 1.06, 95% CI 0.74 to 1.52, p=0.001 for interaction). Patients assigned to the CRT-D arm had significant reduction in LV end diastolic volume index (–26.2 versus –7.4 mL/m²), LV end systolic volume index (–28.7 versus –9.1 mL/m²) as well as improvement in LVEF (11% versus 3%) compared to the ICD only group. After adjusting for baseline variables, for every 10% reduction in the LV end diastolic volume index, there was a 40% reduction in the risk of death or heart failure hospitalization (Solomon et al.). Furthermore MADIT CRT measured echocardiographic response as a decrease in LV end systolic volume > 25%. Using this definition, 529 patients assigned to the CRT-D arm responded to CRT and were less likely to have ventricular tachyarrhythmia (VT or VF) and inappropriate shocks. Analysis of the data showed that for every 10% reduction in LV end systolic volume, there is a 20% decrease in the risk of ventricular tachyarrhythmias (p<0.001) even after adjusting for other clinical risk factors including age, QRS duration, left bundle branch block, and blood urea nitrogen (BUN) (Barsheshet et al.).

The Resynchronization-Defibrillation for Ambulatory Heart Failure Trial (RAFT) randomized 1798 patients with LVEF <30%, NYHA II to III heart failure and QRS duration of >120 msec or a paced QRS duration of > 200 msec to either ICD alone or Biventricular defibrillator (CRT-D) (Tang et al.). Mean follow up was for 40 months and the primary endpoint was death or hospitalization for heart failure while secondary endpoints included death from any cause, death from cardiovascular cause and heart failure hospitalization. Most of the patient had NYHA class II (80%) and had ischemic etiology (64%). Patients with CRT-D had less death and heart failure hospitalization compared to the ICD group (HR 0.75, 95% CI of 0.64 to 0.87, p <0.001). CRT-D also improved survival compared to ICD alone (HR 0.75, 95% CI 0.62-0.91, p=0.003) (Figure 4). There was less heart failure hospitalizations with CRT-D group compared to ICD only group (HR 0.68, 95% CI of 0.56 to 0.83, p<0.001). There was no difference in the primary and secondary endpoints in patients with ischemic and non-ischemic cardiomyopathy. Patients with wider QRS (>150 milliseconds) had better survival than patients with QRS < 150 msec. However, patients with CRT-D had more 30 days adverse events compared to the ICD alone group (p<0.001), these were mostly device related complications.

These trails established CRT as an important therapy for patients with heart failure, LVEF < 35% and NYHA class III to IV. The only measure of dys-synchrony that stood the test of time is the QRS duration. Even though there is disagreement in the literature in the measurement of "response". At least two thirds of patients with CRT show clinical improvement in their functional status. CRT has been proven to improve survival independently as shown in the CARE HF trial, and it also improves survival above and beyond ICD therapy as shown in the RAFT trial. The guidelines for implantation for CRT in patients with systolic heart failure are listed in Table 5. These guidelines were written in 2008, and do not reflect the recent evidence of the benefits of CRT in milder forms of heart failure that was found in the REVERSE, MADIT CRT and RAFT trials.

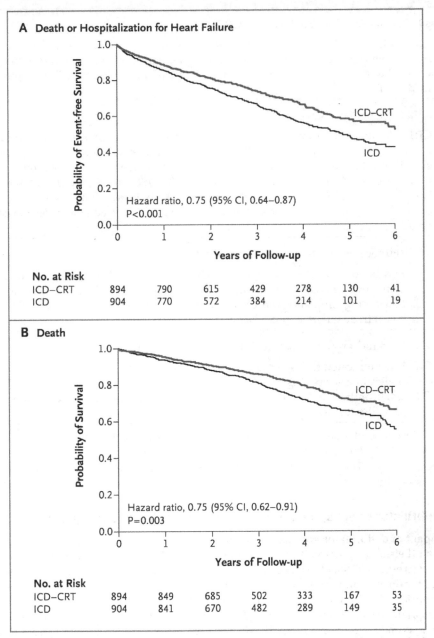

Fig. 4. Kaplan Meier Estimates of Death or Hospitalization for Heart Failure (Panel A) and Death from Any Cause (Panel B). (From Tang, A. S., Wells, G. A., Talajic, M., et al. "Cardiac-resynchronization therapy for mild-to-moderate heart failure." New England Journal of Medicine Vol. 363, No.25, (December, 2010): pp. 2385-2395, ISSN 1533-4406, with permission)

Class I (General agreement of benefit of CRT)
1. CRT with or without an ICD is indicated for the treatment of for patients are in sinus rhythm who have LVEF ≤ 35%, a QRS duration ≥ 120 milliseconds, NYHA functional Class III or ambulatory Class IV heart failure symptoms with optimal recommended medical therapy.
Class IIa (Weight of evidence is in favor of CRT)
1. CRT with or without an ICD is indicated for patients in sinus rhythm who have LVEF ≤ 35%, a QRS duration ≥ 120 msec, NYHA functional class III or ambulatory class IV heart failure symptoms with optimal recommended medical therapy. 2. CRT is reasonable for patients with LVEF ≤ 35%, QRS duration ≥120 milliseconds, NYHA functional Class III or ambulatory Class IV heart failure symptoms with optimal recommended medical therapy and who have frequent dependence on ventricular pacing.
Class IIb (Efficacy of CRT is less well established)
1. CRT may be considered for patients with LVEF ≤ 35% with NYHA functional Class I or II symptoms who are receiving optimal recommended medical therapy and who are undergoing implantation of a permanent pacemaker and/or ICD with anticipated frequent ventricular pacing.
Class III (General agreement that CRT is less effective and might be harmful)
1. CRT is not indicated for asymptomatic patients with reduced LVEF in the absence of other indications for pacing. 2. CRT is not indicated for patients whose functional status and life expectancy are limited predominantly by chronic non-cardiac conditions.

Table 5. Recommendations for cardiac resynchronization therapy based on the ACC/AHA/HRS 2008 Guidelines for Device Based Therapy. CRT: Cardiac Resynchronization Therapy. ICD: Implantable Cardioverter Defibrillator. NYHA: New York Heart Association

5. Defibrillator shocks, their impact on quality of life and prognosis

5.1 Impact of defibrillator shocks on quality of life

From all the studies presented earlier, it is clear that ICD therapy prevents sudden cardiac death. However, ICD shocks can be painful and have been shown to affect the quality of life in both primary and secondary prevention trials. Patients with ICD can receive inappropriate shocks due to atrial fibrillation (AF), supraventricular tachycardia (SVT) or inappropriate sensing from the device. The quality of life (QOL) was assessed in the AVID trial as a secondary endpoint using the Medical Outcomes Short Form 36 item questionnaire (SF-36). Of the 905 patients enrolled in QOL analysis, 800 survived for longer than 1 year. Both treatment groups (ICD group versus antiarrhythmic group) had significant impairment in both physical functioning and mental well-being(Schron et al. 2002). ICD shocks were independently associated with reduction in both physical functioning and mental well-being. The CIDS trial also measured QOL, in the 400 patients who survived for

> 1 year, patients assigned to the ICD group had an improvement in their quality of life scores compared to patients assigned to amiodarone. However, patients having frequent shocks (>5 shocks) had reduced QOL.

The SCD-HeFT trial also collected data on the quality of life using two different scales: The Duke Activity Scale Index (DASI) reflecting the overall physical functioning and the SF-36 Mental Health Inventory 5 which measures psychological well being (Mark et al. 2008). Data were collected at baseline, 3, 12 and 30 months of follow up. A total of 2479 patients (98%) enrolled in SCD-HeFT completed the quality of life portion of the study. Patients receiving ICD therapy and patients assigned to placebo had similar DASI scores and SF-36 MHI 5 scores at baseline. The psychological well being of patients receiving an ICD was significantly better at 3 months and 12 months compared to patients receiving placebo. There was no difference in the physical functioning at baseline or at 3, 12 or 30 months in the ICD group versus the placebo group. The quality of life of patients who received an ICD shock a month before the screening was significantly worse in multiple aspects (physical, psychological, social and self related health).

5.2 Impact of defibrillator shocks on prognosis

The SCD-HeFT Trial also evaluated the prognostic impact of ICD shocks in patients with ischemic and non-ischemic cardiomyopathy. Most of the patients received a single chamber ICD programmed to shock only therapy with no antitachycardia pacing involved. (Poole et al. 2008). Patients (n=811) were followed for 45.5 months and a third of patients (n=269) received ICD shocks. Patients who received appropriate ICD shock (n=128) were at increased risk of death (HR 5.68, 95% CI of 3.97 to 8.12, p < 0.001) compared to patients with no appropriate shocks. Patients who received inappropriate shocks were also at increased risk of death (HR 1.98, 95% CI of 1.29 to 3.05, p=0.002) compared to patients with no inappropriate shocks. Atrial fibrillation was the most common reason for inappropriate ICD shocks and the most common cause of death in patients receiving any shock was progressive heart failure.

Inappropriate shocks were examined in the MADIT-II trial. Of the 719 patients who received an ICD, inappropriate shocks occurred in 83 patients (11.5%). Inappropriate shocks represented a third (31.2%) of total shocks (Daubert et al. 2008). Independent predictors of inappropriate shocks included atrial fibrillation (HR = 2.9, P<0.01), smoking (HR 2.18, P=0.03), diastolic blood pressure of > 80 mmHg (HR = 1.61, P= 0.04) and antecedent appropriate shocks (HR = 2.25, P= 0.03). Again, inappropriate shocks were most likely due to AF (44%), SVT (36%) or abnormal sensing (20%). Implantation of a dual chamber ICD did not decrease the rate of inappropriate shocks compared to single chamber ICD implantation (38.6% versus 44% respectively, p=0.31). Any shock whether appropriate or inappropriate was associated with significant increase in mortality (HR 4.08, p<0.01). Inappropriate shocks were associated with a 2 fold increase in mortality (HR is 2.29, p=0.03) while appropriate shocks had a 3 fold increase in mortality (HR 3.36, p<0.01). Electrical instability in the form of VT or VF or atrial fibrillation could be markers of deteriorating heart function and pump failure(Obadah Al Chekakie 2009). It is unclear if the VT or VF that the patient experiences heralds progressive pump failure, or whether the fact that shocks my increase mortality due to their negative effect on contractility in this high risk population or if both assumptions are true.

5.3 Device programming studies: Safety, effectiveness and impact on quality of life

Since Shocks are associated with lower quality of life and increase mortality, attempts at reducing shocks (both appropriate and inappropriate) became the focus of several studies. Antitachycardia pacing (ATP) has been shown to terminate 78 to 94% of slow VTs (188 bpm) (Peinado et al. 1998). The PAINFREE RX II trial randomized 634 patients with ICDs to standardized ATP (n=313 patients) versus shocks (n=321 patients). The programming in the Standarized ATP arm included two main parameters: First programming ATP in the fast VT zone of 188 to 250 bpm, at 8 pulses and 88% of VT cycle length. Second is extending the detection to 18 of 24 beats to avoid shocking ventricular tachycardia that was going to terminate anyway. The primary objective was to demonstrate that ATP will not prolong treatment > 6 seconds compared to the shock arm. Secondary objectives included the QOL, ATP efficacy and acceleration and syncope (Sweeney et al. 2005). After mean follow up of 11+/- 3 months, 4230 ICD counters were retrieved, and electrograms were only available in 1827 episodes. A third of the shocks was deemed inappropriate and due to SVT and 0.2% were due to noise. Only 73% of total shocks were due to true ventricular arrhythmias. Of these, 431 (58%) were detected as VT, 32% as Fast VT and 10% as VF. ATP was successful as initial therapy in 81% of the episodes and failed in 54 episodes, of which 49 episodes were shocked while 5 were terminated by a second ATP therapy. ATP did not prolong therapy duration (median duration was 10 seconds in the ATP arm versus 9.7 seconds in the shock arm) and there was no significant difference in the acceleration of VT/VF between the two arms. Syncope was very rare in the two arms (2 in the ATP group and 1 in the shock arm) and the first shock success was identical between the two arms. There was no difference between the two groups at baseline in the QOL scores as assessed by the SF-36. Patients assigned to the shock arm had an improvement in the bodily pain scores at 12 months but no change in the other SF-36 subscales. While patients assigned to the ATP arm had significant improvement in 5 subscales (bodily pain, social functioning, role emotional, physical functioning and role physical). This trial established the safety and efficacy of ATP in the fast VT zone and the safety of extending the detection duration to 18 out of 24 beats, which led to a decrease in shocks (The patients assigned to the shock arm had 147 detected FVT episodes with only 99 episodes receiving therapy). This will be an important factor in the design and implementation of the PREPARE study.

The Primary Prevention Parameters Evaluation Study (PREPARE) study compared 700 patients who had received an ICD or Biventricular defibrillator for primary prevention within 6 months of enrollment (Wilkoff et al. 2008). The control group for the ICD patients was taken from the EMPIRIC trial while the control group for the Biventricular ICD (BiV ICD) arm was from the MIRACLE ICD trial. The cohort of the PREPARE study had the following programming parameters: Initial detection for VT at rate of >182 bpm, with ATP programmed to fast VT of 182 to 250 bpm, with detection prolonged to 30 of the 40 intervals to avoid shocking VT that was going to terminate anyway, programming SVT discriminators to arrhythmias < 200 bpm to prevent inappropriate shocks. The primary endpoint of the study was the morbidity index defined as 1) device related cardioversion or defibrillation whether appropriate or inappropriate, 2) syncope secondary to arrhythmia or presumed arrhythmia and 3) untreated sustained symptomatic VT/VF events. The PREPARE study patients were less likely to receive a shock for any cause in the first year as compared to the control cohort (8.5 % vs 16.9%, p<0.01) and were also less likely to receive inappropriate shocks even after correcting for differences in baseline variables including mean LVEF, hypertension, history of ischemic heart disease, syncope and baseline use of beta blockers. The morbidity index incidence density was significantly lower in the PREPARE cohort compared to the control cohorts (HR 0.26 versus 0.69, 95% CI of 0.2 to 0.72, p=0.003). Importantly, only 12 of the 40 syncope episodes were judged to be due to arrhythmia, and of those, only 11 were due to PREPARE programming. The PREPARE study established the efficacy of empirically programming the ICD detection and therapy to minimize both appropriate and inappropriate shocks. This is true for patients receiving ICD therapy for primary prevention only.

In summary: ICD therapy prevents sudden cardiac death but patients who receive an ICD shock have increased morbidity and mortality and poor quality of life. Programming the device can help minimize ICD shocks, whether appropriate or inappropriate. Patients with ICD therapy who receive a shock should be followed closely since they are at increased risk of pump failure.

6. Conclusion

Implantable cardioverter defibrillator therapy is important in sudden cardiac death prevention in patients with ischemic and non-ischemic cardiomyopathy as well as survivors of cardiac arrest. Cardiac resynchronization therapy with and without an ICD improves the quality of life and leads to reverse remodeling and independently prevents sudden cardiac death in patients with QRS > 120 msec and LVEF < 35% who are on optimal medical therapy. Defibrillator shocks are associated with adverse outcomes and pump failure. Careful patient selection and sophisticated programming can help prevent sudden cardiac death without compromising the quality of life of the patients.

7. References

Abraham, W. T., Fisher, W. G., Smith, A. L., et al. (2002). "Cardiac resynchronization in chronic heart failure." *New England Journal of Medicine* Vol. 346, No.24, (June, 2002): pp. 1845-1853, ISSN: 1533-4406

Arshad, A., Moss, A. J., Foster, E., et al. "Cardiac resynchronization therapy is more effective in women than in men: the MADIT-CRT (Multicenter Automatic Defibrillator Implantation Trial with Cardiac Resynchronization Therapy) trial." *Journal of The American College of Cardiology* Vol. 57, No.7, (February, 2011): pp. 813-820, ISSN 1558-3597

AVID Investigators (1997). "A comparison of antiarrhythmic-drug therapy with implantable defibrillators in patients resuscitated from near-fatal ventricular arrhythmias. The Antiarrhythmics versus Implantable Defibrillators (AVID) Investigators." *New England Journal of Medicine* Vol. 337, No.22, (November, 1997): pp. 1576-1583, ISSN 0028-4793

Bardy, G. H., Lee, K. L., Mark, D. B., et al. (2005). "Amiodarone or an implantable cardioverter-defibrillator for congestive heart failure." *New England Journal of Medicine* Vol. 352, No.3, (January, 2005): pp. 225-237, ISSN 1533-4406

Barsheshet, A., Wang, P. J., Moss, A. J., et al. "Reverse Remodeling and the Risk of Ventricular Tachyarrhythmias in the MADIT-CRT (Multicenter Automatic Defibrillator Implantation Trial-Cardiac Resynchronization Therapy)." *Journal of*

The American College of Cardiology Vol. 57, No.24, (June, 2011): pp. 2416-2423, ISSN 1558-3597

Beshai, J. F., Grimm, R. A., Nagueh, S. F., et al. (2007). "Cardiac-resynchronization therapy in heart failure with narrow QRS complexes." *New England Journal of Medicine* Vol. 357, No.24, (December, 2007): pp. 2461-2471, ISSN 1533-4406

Bigger, J. T., Jr. (1997). "Prophylactic use of implanted cardiac defibrillators in patients at high risk for ventricular arrhythmias after coronary-artery bypass graft surgery. Coronary Artery Bypass Graft (CABG) Patch Trial Investigators." *New England Journal of Medicine* Vol. 337, No.22, (November, 1997): pp. 1569-1575, ISSN 0028-4793

Blanc, J. J., Etienne, Y., Gilard, M., et al. (1997). "Evaluation of different ventricular pacing sites in patients with severe heart failure: results of an acute hemodynamic study." *Circulation* Vol. 96, No.10, (November, 1997): pp. 3273-3277, ISSN 0009-7322

Bristow, M. R., Saxon, L. A., Boehmer, J., et al. (2004). "Cardiac-resynchronization therapy with or without an implantable defibrillator in advanced chronic heart failure." *New England Journal of Medicine* Vol. 350, No.21, (May, 2004): pp. 2140-2150, ISSN 1533-4406

Buxton, A. E., Lee, K. L., DiCarlo, L., et al. (2000). "Electrophysiologic testing to identify patients with coronary artery disease who are at risk for sudden death. Multicenter Unsustained Tachycardia Trial Investigators." *New England Journal of Medicine* Vol. 342, No.26, (June, 2000): pp. 1937-1945, ISSN 0028-4793

Buxton, A. E., Lee, K. L., Fisher, J. D., et al. (1999). "A randomized study of the prevention of sudden death in patients with coronary artery disease. Multicenter Unsustained Tachycardia Trial Investigators." *New England Journal of Medicin* Vol. 341, No.25, (December, 1999): pp. 1882-1890, ISSN 0028-4793

Chung, E. S., Leon, A. R., Tavazzi, L., et al. (2008). "Results of the Predictors of Response to CRT (PROSPECT) trial." *Circulation* Vol. 117, No.20, (May, 2008): pp. 2608-2616, ISSN 1524-4539

Cleland, J. G., Daubert, J. C., Erdmann, E., et al. (2005). "The effect of cardiac resynchronization on morbidity and mortality in heart failure." *New England Journal of Medicine* Vol. 352, No.15, (April, 2005): pp. 1539-1549, ISSN 1533-4406

Connolly, S. J., Gent, M., Roberts, R. S., et al. (2000). "Canadian implantable defibrillator study (CIDS) : a randomized trial of the implantable cardioverter defibrillator against amiodarone." *Circulation* Vol. 101, No.11, (March, 2000): pp. 1297-1302, ISSN 1524-4539

Connolly, S. J., Hallstrom, A. P., Cappato, R., et al. (2000). "Meta-analysis of the implantable cardioverter defibrillator secondary prevention trials. AVID, CASH and CIDS studies. Antiarrhythmics vs Implantable Defibrillator study. Cardiac Arrest Study Hamburg . Canadian Implantable Defibrillator Study." *European Heart Journal* Vol. 21, No.24, (December, 2000): pp. 2071-2078, ISSN 0195-668X

Corrado, D., Leoni, L., Link, M. S., et al. (2003). "Implantable cardioverter-defibrillator therapy for prevention of sudden death in patients with arrhythmogenic right ventricular cardiomyopathy/dysplasia." *Circulation* Vol. 108, No.25, (December, 2003): pp. 3084-3091, ISSN 1524-4539

Daubert, J. P., Zareba, W., Cannom, D. S., et al. (2008). "Inappropriate implantable cardioverter-defibrillator shocks in MADIT II: frequency, mechanisms, predictors, and survival impact." *Journal of The American College of Cardiology* Vol. 51, No.14, (April, 2008): pp. 1357-1365, ISSN 1558-3597

Daubert, J. P., Zareba, W., Hall, W. J., et al. (2006). "Predictive value of ventricular arrhythmia inducibility for subsequent ventricular tachycardia or ventricular fibrillation in Multicenter Automatic Defibrillator Implantation Trial (MADIT) II patients." *Journal of The American College of Cardiology* Vol. 47, No.1, (January, 2006): pp. 98-107, ISSN 1558-3597

Domanski, M. J., Exner, D. V., Borkowf, C. B., et al. (1999). "Effect of angiotensin converting enzyme inhibition on sudden cardiac death in patients following acute myocardial infarction. A meta-analysis of randomized clinical trials." *Journal of The American College of Cardiology* Vol. 33, No.3, (March, 1999): pp. 598-604, ISSN 0735-1097

Domanski, M. J., Sakseena, S., Epstein, A. E., et al. (1999). "Relative effectiveness of the implantable cardioverter-defibrillator and antiarrhythmic drugs in patients with varying degrees of left ventricular dysfunction who have survived malignant ventricular arrhythmias. AVID Investigators. Antiarrhythmics Versus Implantable Defibrillators." *Journal of The American College of Cardiology* Vol. 34, No.4, (October, 1999): pp. 1090-1095, ISSN 0735-1097

Epstein, A. E., DiMarco, J. P., Ellenbogen, K. A., et al. (2008). "ACC/AHA/HRS 2008 Guidelines for Device-Based Therapy of Cardiac Rhythm Abnormalities: a report of the American College of Cardiology/American Heart Association Task Force on Practice Guidelines (Writing Committee to Revise the ACC/AHA/NASPE 2002 Guideline Update for Implantation of Cardiac Pacemakers and Antiarrhythmia Devices): developed in collaboration with the American Association for Thoracic Surgery and Society of Thoracic Surgeons." *Circulation* Vol. 117, No.21, (May, 2008): pp. e350-408, ISSN 1524-4539

Fornwalt, B. K., Sprague, W. W., BeDell, P., et al. "Agreement is poor among current criteria used to define response to cardiac resynchronization therapy." *Circulation* Vol. 121, No.18, (May, 2010): pp. 1985-1991, ISSN 1524-4539

Gemayel, C., Pelliccia, A. and Thompson, P. D. (2001). "Arrhythmogenic right ventricular cardiomyopathy." *Journal of The American College of Cardiology* Vol. 38, No.7, (December, 2001): pp. 1773-1781, ISSN 0735-1097

Goldenberg, I., Moss, A. J., McNitt, S., et al. (2006). "Time dependence of defibrillator benefit after coronary revascularization in the Multicenter Automatic Defibrillator Implantation Trial (MADIT)-II." *Journal of The American College of Cardiology* Vol. 47, No.9, (May, 2006): pp. 1811-1817, ISSN 1558-3597

Gorgels, A. P., Gijsbers, C., de Vreede-Swagemakers, J., et al. (2003). "Out-of-hospital cardiac arrest--the relevance of heart failure. The Maastricht Circulatory Arrest Registry." *European Heart Journal* Vol. 24, No.13, (July, 2003): pp. 1204-1209, ISSN 0195-668X

Higgins, S. L., Hummel, J. D., Niazi, I. K., et al. (2003). "Cardiac resynchronization therapy for the treatment of heart failure in patients with intraventricular conduction delay and malignant ventricular tachyarrhythmias." *Journal of The American College of Cardiology* Vol. 42, No.8, (October, 2003): pp. 1454-1459, ISSN 0735-1097

Hohnloser, S. H., Kuck, K. H., Dorian, P., et al. (2004). "Prophylactic use of an implantable cardioverter-defibrillator after acute myocardial infarction." *New England Journal of Medicine* Vol. 351, No.24, (December9, 2004): pp. 2481-2488, ISSN 1533-4406

Hulot, J. S., Jouven, X., Empana, J. P., et al. (2004). "Natural history and risk stratification of arrhythmogenic right ventricular dysplasia/cardiomyopathy." *Circulation* Vol. 110, No.14, (October, 2004): pp. 1879-1884, ISSN 1524-4539

Kadish, A., Dyer, A., Daubert, J. P., et al. (2004). "Prophylactic defibrillator implantation in patients with nonischemic dilated cardiomyopathy." *New England Journal of Medicine* Vol. 350, No.21, (May, 2004): pp. 2151-2158, ISSN 1533-4406

Kadish, A., Schaechter, A., Subacius, H., et al. (2006). "Patients with recently diagnosed nonischemic cardiomyopathy benefit from implantable cardioverter-defibrillators." *Journal of The American College of Cardiology* Vol. 47, No.12, (June, 2006): pp. 2477-2482, ISSN 1558-3597

Kofflard, M. J., Ten Cate, F. J., van der Lee, C., et al. (2003). "Hypertrophic cardiomyopathy in a large community-based population: clinical outcome and identification of risk factors for sudden cardiac death and clinical deterioration." *Journal of The American College of Cardiology* Vol. 41, No.6, (March, 2003): pp. 987-993, ISSN 0735-1097

Kuck, K. H., Cappato, R., Siebels, J., et al. (2000). "Randomized comparison of antiarrhythmic drug therapy with implantable defibrillators in patients resuscitated from cardiac arrest : the Cardiac Arrest Study Hamburg (CASH)." *Circulation* Vol. 102, No.7, (August, 2000): pp. 748-754, ISSN 1524-4539

Leclercq, J. F., Potenza, S., Maison-Blanche, P., et al. (1996). "Determinants of spontaneous occurrence of sustained monomorphic ventricular tachycardia in right ventricular dysplasia." *Journal of The American College of Cardiology* Vol. 28, No.3, (September, 1996): pp. 720-724, ISSN 0735-1097

Linde, C., Abraham, W. T., Gold, M. R., et al. (2008). "Randomized trial of cardiac resynchronization in mildly symptomatic heart failure patients and in asymptomatic patients with left ventricular dysfunction and previous heart failure symptoms." *Journal of The American College of Cardiology* Vol. 52, No.23, (December, 2008): pp. 1834-1843, ISSN 1558-3597

Marcus, G. M., Glidden, D. V., Polonsky, B., et al. (2009). "Efficacy of antiarrhythmic drugs in arrhythmogenic right ventricular cardiomyopathy: a report from the North American ARVC Registry." *Journal of The American College of Cardiology* Vol. 54, No.7, (August, 2009): pp. 609-615, ISSN 1558-3597

Mark, D. B., Anstrom, K. J., Sun, J. L., et al. (2008). "Quality of life with defibrillator therapy or amiodarone in heart failure." *New England Journal of Medicine* Vol. 359, No.10, (September, 2008): pp. 999-1008, ISSN 1533-4406

Mark, D. B., Nelson, C. L., Anstrom, K. J., et al. (2006). "Cost-effectiveness of defibrillator therapy or amiodarone in chronic stable heart failure: results from the Sudden Cardiac Death in Heart Failure Trial (SCD-HeFT)." *Circulation* Vol. 114, No.2, (July, 2006): pp. 135-142, ISSN 1524-4539

Maron, B. J. (2002). "Hypertrophic cardiomyopathy: a systematic review." *Journal of the American Medical Association* Vol. 287, No.10, (March, 2002): pp. 1308-1320, ISSN 0098-7484

Maron, B. J. (2003). "Sudden death in young athletes." *New England Journal of Medicine* Vol. 349, No.11, (September, 2003): pp. 1064-1075, ISSN 1533-4406

Maron, B. J., Casey, S. A., Poliac, L. C., et al. (1999). "Clinical course of hypertrophic cardiomyopathy in a regional United States cohort." *Journal of the American Medical Association* Vol. 281, No.7, (February, 1999): pp. 650-655, ISSN 0098-7484

Maron, B. J., McKenna, W. J., Danielson, G. K., et al. (2003). "American College of Cardiology/European Society of Cardiology clinical expert consensus document on hypertrophic cardiomyopathy. A report of the American College of Cardiology Foundation Task Force on Clinical Expert Consensus Documents and the European Society of Cardiology Committee for Practice Guidelines." *Journal of The American College of Cardiology* Vol. 42, No.9, (November, 2003): pp. 1687-1713, ISSN 0735-1097 (

Maron, B. J., Shen, W. K., Link, M. S., et al. (2000). "Efficacy of implantable cardioverter-defibrillators for the prevention of sudden death in patients with hypertrophic cardiomyopathy." *New England Journal of Medicine* Vol. 342, No.6, (February, 2000): pp. 365-373, ISSN 0028-4793

Maron, B. J., Spirito, P., Shen, W. K., et al. (2007). "Implantable cardioverter-defibrillators and prevention of sudden cardiac death in hypertrophic cardiomyopathy."*Journal of the American Medical Association* Vol. 298, No.4, (July, 2007): pp. 405-412, ISSN 1538-3598

Maron, B. J., Wolfson, J. K., Epstein, S. E., et al. (1986). "Intramural ("small vessel") coronary artery disease in hypertrophic cardiomyopathy." *Journal of The American College of Cardiology* Vol. 8, No.3, (September, 1986): pp. 545-557, ISSN 0735-1097

Maron, M. S., Olivotto, I., Betocchi, S., et al. (2003). "Effect of left ventricular outflow tract obstruction on clinical outcome in hypertrophic cardiomyopathy." *New England Journal of Medicine* Vol. 348, No.4, (January, 2003): pp. 295-303, ISSN 1533-4406

McKenna, W. J., Thiene, G., Nava, A., et al. (1994). "Diagnosis of arrhythmogenic right ventricular dysplasia/cardiomyopathy. Task Force of the Working Group Myocardial and Pericardial Disease of the European Society of Cardiology and of the Scientific Council on Cardiomyopathies of the International Society and Federation of Cardiology." *British Heart* Journal Vol. 71, No.3, (March, 1994): pp. 215-218, ISSN 0007-0769

McMurray, J., Kober, L., Robertson, M., et al. (2005). "Antiarrhythmic effect of carvedilol after acute myocardial infarction: results of the Carvedilol Post-Infarct Survival Control in Left Ventricular Dysfunction (CAPRICORN) trial." *Journal of The American College of Cardiology* Vol. 45, No.4, (Febrary, 2005): pp. 525-530, ISSN 0735-1097

Moss, A. J., Hall, W. J., Cannom, D. S., et al. (1996). "Improved survival with an implanted defibrillator in patients with coronary disease at high risk for ventricular arrhythmia. Multicenter Automatic Defibrillator Implantation Trial Investigators." *New England Journal of Medicine* Vol. 335, No.26, (December, 1996): pp. 1933-1940, ISSN 0028-4793

Moss, A. J., Hall, W. J., Cannom, D. S., et al. (2009). "Cardiac-resynchronization therapy for the prevention of heart-failure events." *New England Journal of Medicien* Vol. 361, No.14, (October, 2009): pp. 1329-1338, ISSN 1533-4406

Moss, A. J., Zareba, W., Hall, W. J., et al. (2002). "Prophylactic implantation of a defibrillator in patients with myocardial infarction and reduced ejection fraction." *New England Journal of Medicine* Vol. 346, No.12, (March, 2002): pp. 877-883, ISSN 1533-4406

Nanthakumar, K., Epstein, A. E., Kay, G. N., et al. (2004). "Prophylactic implantable cardioverter-defibrillator therapy in patients with left ventricular systolic dysfunction: a pooled analysis of 10 primary prevention trials." *Journal of The American College of Cardiology* Vol. 44, No.11, (December, 2004): pp. 2166-2172, ISSN 0735-1097

Nelson, G. S., Curry, C. W., Wyman, B. T., et al. (2000). "Predictors of systolic augmentation from left ventricular preexcitation in patients with dilated cardiomyopathy and intraventricular conduction delay." *Circulation* Vol. 101, No.23, (June, 2000): pp. 2703-2709, ISSN 1524-4539

O'Brien, B. J., Connolly, S. J., Goeree, R., et al. (2001). "Cost-effectiveness of the implantable cardioverter-defibrillator: results from the Canadian Implantable Defibrillator Study (CIDS)." *Circulation* Vol. 103, No.10, (March, 2001): pp. 1416-1421, ISSN 1524-4539

Al Chekakie, M. (2009). "Electrical instability heralding worsening heart failure in a patient with nonischemic dilated cardiomyopathy." *Congestive Heart Failure* Vol. 15, No.5, (September, 2009): pp. 249-251, ISSN 1751-7133

Peinado, R., Almendral, J., Rius, T., et al. (1998). "Randomized, prospective comparison of four burst pacing algorithms for spontaneous ventricular tachycardia." *American Journal of Cardiology* Vol. 82, No.11, (December, 1998): pp. 1422-1425, A1428-1429, ISSN 0002-9149

Pitt, B., Remme, W., Zannad, F., et al. (2003). "Eplerenone, a selective aldosterone blocker, in patients with left ventricular dysfunction after myocardial infarction." *New England Journal of Medicine* Vol. 348, No.14, (April, 2003): pp. 1309-1321, ISSN 1533-4406

Poole, J. E., Johnson, G. W., Hellkamp, A. S., et al. (2008). "Prognostic importance of defibrillator shocks in patients with heart failure." *New England Journal of Medicine* Vol. 359, No.10, (September, 2008): pp. 1009-1017, ISSN 1533-4406

Roguin, A., Bomma, C. S., Nasir, K., et al. (2004). "Implantable cardioverter-defibrillators in patients with arrhythmogenic right ventricular dysplasia/cardiomyopathy." *Journal of The American College of Cardiology* Vol. 43, No.10, (May, 2004): pp. 1843-1852, ISSN 0735-1097

Sanders, G. D., Hlatky, M. A. and Owens, D. K. (2005). "Cost-effectiveness of implantable cardioverter-defibrillators." *New England Journal of Medicine* Vol. 353, No.14, (October, 2005): pp. 1471-1480, ISSN 1533-4406

Schron, E. B., Exner, D. V., Yao, Q., et al. (2002). "Quality of life in the antiarrhythmics versus implantable defibrillators trial: impact of therapy and influence of adverse symptoms and defibrillator shocks." *Circulation* Vol. 105, No.5, (February, 2002): pp. 589-594, ISSN 1524-4539

Seidl, K., Hauer, B., Schwick, N. G., et al. (1998). "Comparison of metoprolol and sotalol in preventing ventricular tachyarrhythmias after the implantation of a cardioverter/defibrillator." *American Journal of Cardiology* Vol. 82, No.6, (September, 1998): pp. 744-748, ISSN 0002-9149

Sen-Chowdhry, S., Lowe, M. D., Sporton, S. C., et al. (2004). "Arrhythmogenic right ventricular cardiomyopathy: clinical presentation, diagnosis, and management." *American Journal of Medicine* Vol. 117, No.9, (November, 2004): pp. 685-695, ISSN 0002-9343

Solomon, S. D., Foster, E., Bourgoun, M., et al. "Effect of cardiac resynchronization therapy on reverse remodeling and relation to outcome: multicenter automatic defibrillator implantation trial: cardiac resynchronization therapy." *Circulation* Vol. 122, No.10, (September: pp. 985-992, ISSN 1524-4539

Steinbeck, G., Andresen, D., Seidl, K., et al. (2009). "Defibrillator implantation early after myocardial infarction." *New England Journal of Medicine* Vol. 361, No.15, (October, 2009): pp. 1427-1436, ISSN 1533-4406

Sweeney, M. O., Wathen, M. S., Volosin, K., et al. (2005). "Appropriate and inappropriate ventricular therapies, quality of life, and mortality among primary and secondary prevention implantable cardioverter defibrillator patients: results from the Pacing Fast VT REduces Shock ThErapies (PainFREE Rx II) trial." *Circulation* Vol. 111, No.22, (June 7, 2005): pp. 2898-2905, ISSN 1524-4539

Tabib, A., Loire, R., Chalabreysse, L., et al. (2003). "Circumstances of death and gross and microscopic observations in a series of 200 cases of sudden death associated with arrhythmogenic right ventricular cardiomyopathy and/or dysplasia." *Circulation* Vol. 108, No.24, (December, 2003): pp. 3000-3005, ISSN 1524-4539

Tang, A. S., Wells, G. A., Talajic, M., et al. "Cardiac-resynchronization therapy for mild-to-moderate heart failure." *New England Journal of Medicine* Vol. 363, No.25, (December, 2010: pp. 2385-2395, ISSN 1533-4406

Varnava, A. M., Elliott, P. M., Mahon, N., et al. (2001). "Relation between myocyte disarray and outcome in hypertrophic cardiomyopathy." *American Journal of Cardiology* Vol. 88, No.3, (August, 2001): pp. 275-279, ISSN 0002-9149

Veenhuyzen, G. D., Singh, S. N., McAreavey, D., et al. (2001). "Prior coronary artery bypass surgery and risk of death among patients with ischemic left ventricular dysfunction." *Circulation* Vol. 104, No.13, (September, 2001): pp. 1489-1493, ISSN 1524-4539

Wilber, D. J., Zareba, W., Hall, W. J., et al. (2004). "Time dependence of mortality risk and defibrillator benefit after myocardial infarction." *Circulation* Vol. 109, No.9, (March, 2004): pp. 1082-1084, ISSN 1524-4539

Wilkoff, B. L., Williamson, B. D., Stern, R. S., et al. (2008). "Strategic programming of detection and therapy parameters in implantable cardioverter-defibrillators reduces shocks in primary prevention patients: results from the PREPARE (Primary Prevention Parameters Evaluation) study." *Journal of The American College of Cardiology* Vol. 52, No.7, (August 12, 2008): pp. 541-550, ISSN 1558-3597

Wyse, D. G., Friedman, P. L., Brodsky, M. A., et al. (2001). "Life-threatening ventricular arrhythmias due to transient or correctable causes: high risk for death in follow-up." *Journal of The American College of Cardiology* Vol. 38, No.6, (November, 2001): pp. 1718-1724, ISSN 0735-1097

Young, J. B., Abraham, W. T., Smith, A. L., et al. (2003). "Combined cardiac resynchronization and implantable cardioversion defibrillation in advanced chronic heart failure: the MIRACLE ICD Trial." *JAMA* Vol. 289, No.20, (May, 2003): pp. 2685-2694, ISSN 0098-7484

Zipes, D. P., Camm, A. J., Borggrefe, M., et al. (2006). "ACC/AHA/ESC 2006 guidelines for management of patients with ventricular arrhythmias and the prevention of sudden cardiac death: a report of the American College of Cardiology/American Heart Association Task Force and the European Society of Cardiology Committee for Practice Guidelines (Writing Committee to Develop Guidelines for Management of Patients With Ventricular Arrhythmias and the Prevention of Sudden Cardiac Death)." *Journal of The American College of Cardiology* Vol. 48, No.5, (September, 2006): pp. e247-346, ISSN 1558-3597

4

Biomarker for Cardiomyopathy-B-Type Natriuretic Peptide

Mototsugu Nishii and Tohru Izumi
Kitasato University School of Medicine
Japan

1. Introduction

Cardiomyopathy is cardiac condition in which the normal muscular function of the myocardium has been altered by a variety of etiologies. Atherosclerotic coronary artery disease is the most common cause of cardiomyopathy in North America and Europe. Idiopathic cardiomyopathy is the second most common cause, although this may partially include undiagnosed etiologies such as viral infection, drug toxicity, and genetic factors. Other causes include endocrine diseases, collagen vascular diseases, metabolic disorders (hemochromatosis, amyloidosis, glycogen storage disease), neuromuscular disorders, and granulomatous diseases (sarcoidosis).

The cardiac malfunctions are variable, namely left ventricular (LV) systolic dysfunction, LV diastolic dysfunction, or both in accordance with etiologies and morphological findings (cardiac hypertrophy or dilatation). For example, hypertrophic cardiomyopathy initially has LV diastolic dysfunction, while amyloidosis that shows similar morphological change has LV systolic dysfunction. Ischemic or idiopathic cardiomyopathy with ventricular dilatation is represented by systolic dysfunction. Cardiac malfunctions are also altered on disease course. Initially, patients with cardiomyopathy may have asymptomatic LV systolic or diastolic dysfunction alone. However, adverse disease processes finally lead to both dysfunctions.

Imbalance between cardiac malfunctions and compensatory mechanisms worsens an outcome of cardiomyopathy. When abnormal LV filling pressure and volume is unable to be compensated by hemodynamic alterations such as the increases in heart rate and peripheral vascular tone by the accelerated vasoconstrictors including norepinephrine (NE), endothelin-1 (ET-1), and the renin-angiotensin-aldosterone (RAA), this imbalance precipitates decompensated heart failure (HF).

Early and simply identifying the decompensatory process is important therapeutic strategy in cardiomyopathy. Clinical utility of B-type natriuretic peptide (BNP) sensitively produced and secreted from heart in response to LV overload has been extended rapidly in patients with HF. At first, BNP emerged as a diagnostic marker for decompensated HF. Furthermore, BNP has been proved to predict a subsequent outcome in patients with HF. Recently, the efficiency of BNP-guided therapy in patients with HF has been demonstrated. In this chapter, we discuss about clinical utility of BNP assessments in patients with cardiomyopathy.

2. B-type natriuretic peptide (BNP)

BNP is predominantly secreted from the overloaded LV as a 76 aminoacid N-terminal fragment and a 32 aminoacid active hormone, and synthesis and release of BNP are adversely and rapidly accelerated in conjunction with the degree of LV wall stretch (1-2). In addition to this primary regulation, BNP synthesis can be also upregulated by tachycardia, glucocorticoids, thyroid hormones, vasoactive peptides such as ET-1, angiotensin II, and NE, and inflammatory cytokines. On the other hand, BNP is clearance via the binding to a natriuretic peptide receptor (NPR)-C of three NPRs (NPR-A, -B, -C). BNP is also inactivated by neutral endopeptidase, a zinc metallopeptidase which is expressed on the surface of endothelial cells, smooth-muscle cells, cardiac myocytes, renal epithelium, and fibroblasts.
BNP is included into compensatory mechanisms against HF. BNP promotes glomerular filtration and inhibits sodium reabsorption, resulting in natriuresis and diuresis. It reduces blood pressure through the relaxation of vascular smooth muscle and inhibits activations of not only central and peripheral sympathetic nerve systems but also cardiac sympathetic nervous system (3). Furthermore, it also inhibits the RAA system (4).

2.1 BNP as a diagnostic marker
2.1.1 BNP in heart failure
Plasma BNP levels have proven utility in the diagnostic evaluation of decompensated HF in patients with acute dyspnea (5-6). Particularly, BNP at a cutoff of 100 pg/ml could diagnose HF better than not only all other clinical parameters but also the clinical judgement by the emergency room physicians. However, BNP also has the diagostic limitation for HF. BNP is less accurate in detection of asymptomatic LV dysfunction than clinical parameters, because BNP has a close correlation with New York Heart Association (NYHA) functional class and patients with mild LV dysfunction often show normal range of BNP levels.

2.1.2 BNP in cardiomyopathy
BNP levels are raised in dilated, hypertrophic, and restrictive cardiomyopathies. Its increases seem to be different in accordance with cardiac malfunctions. BNP levels are generally higher in patients with systolic dysfunction than in those with isolated diastolic dysfunction, and highest in those with both dysfunctions (7). Furthermore, among patients with preserved LV systolic function, BNP correlates with the severity of diastolic dysfunction. BNP levels are raised in patients with impaired relaxation and especially highest in those with a restrictive filling pattern (8). BNP measurements may facilitate understanding the type and severity of cardiac malfunction on cardiomyopathy.
On the other hand, BNP measurement may be unavailable for distinguishing cardiomyopathies. Hypertrophic cardiomyopathy often shows extremely high levels of BNP, similarly to dilated cardiomyopathy (9). In addition, restrictive cardiomyopathy with systolic dysfunction also shows higher levels of BNP than that with diastolic dysfunction alone (8). However, several reports have demonstrated that BNP is able to distinguish constrictive pericarditis and restrictive cardiomyopathy, although these diseases overlap signs and symptoms of congestion (10). The level of BNP is elevated in patients with restriction, while level is nearly normal in those with constriction. The absence of cardiac stretch by constricting pericardium is thought to lead to lower BNP release.

2.2 BNP as a prognostic marker
Prognostic values of BNP have been identified in various heart diseases such as HF, cardiovascular diseases, and cardiomyopathy.

2.2.1 Heart failure
In patients with HF, higher levels of BNP have been implicated in increased risk of cardiovascular or all-cause mortality and readmission for decompensated HF. Furthermore, the cutoff points on the risk assessment curve are altered on time course after decompensated HF. In admitted patients for decompensated HF, the cutoff point of 800 pg/ml was associated with the increased risk of in-hospital mortality as shown by the ADHERE (Acute Decompensated Heart Failure National Registry) data (11). After the treatment, the predischarge cutoff point for the risk of readmission and mortality falls to about 500 pg/ml (12). The cutoff point further declined to abut 200 pg/ml in clinically stable outpatients after decompensated HF (13). These obsevations suggested that the therapeutic strategies for HF including a safe hospital discharge and the prevention of readmission or cardiac event may be guided by BNP measurement.

2.2.2 Cardiovascular diseases
In disorders other than HF, BNP also has prognostic value. BNP level is able to identify patients at the high risk group of adverse cardiac remodelling from patients with post-myocardial infarction, independent of age, history of HF, and LV ejection fraction (LVEF) (14). Even in patients with unstable angina alone, increased levels of BNP were associated with an increased risk of death (15). In right ventricular dysfunction resulting from pulmonary hypertension, BNP also provides similar prognostic information. These observations have extended the potential role of BNP measurement to risk stratification of cardiovascular events in patients with and without HF.

2.2.3 Cardiac inflammatory diseases; acute myocarditis
Acute myocarditis is able to be mainly divided into two disease conditions on a basis of clinicopathologic profiles, namely fulminant and non-fulminant myocarditis (16-17). Briefly, fulminant myocarditis is represented by the distinct onset of cardiac symptoms within 2 weeks following flu-like symptoms accompanied by histologically proven active myocarditis according to Dallas criteria and severe circulatory failure requiring high-dose intravenous catecholamines use (>5.0 γ) or mechanical circulatory assist devise, while non-fulminant myocarditis is by the indistinct onset of cardiac symptoms without those. Furthermore, these outcomes are distinguished by each unique clinical course (17). Non-fulminant myocarditis has been implicated in poorer long-term outcome than fulminant cases. A few patients with fulminant myocarditis lapsed into mortality from severely deteriorated circulatory collapse refractory to mechanical circulatory assist use or mechanical complications from its long-term use, including bleeding, infections, sepsis, and multiple organ failure. However, more than 80% of fulminant cases recover completely to an uncomplicated status, with cessation of myocardial inflammation and a generally favorable outcome, provided they are able to overcome poor cardiac condition successfully during acute phase (18). On the other hand, non-fulminant myocarditis without severe circulatory failure is likely to develop to chronic HF derived from dilated cardiomyopathy at chronic phase (16-17). Therefore, simple biomarkers to predict a requirement of mechanical assist devise use, outcome following its use, or the development to cardiomyopathy in patients with acute myocarditis have been sought.

Previously, we related various variables to short-term outcome in patients with fulminant myocarditis (19). In-hospital mortality was extremely higher in patients with fulminant myocarditis than in non-fulminant cases. Especially, extremely increased levels of interleukin-10, a major anti-inflammatory cytokine in serum on admission were associated with short-term outcome including mechanical assist use and in-hospital mortality in patients with acute myocarditis (Figure 1), which might be explained by its inhibitory effect on viral elimination from host. A major pathogenic factor of acute myocarditis and subsequent cardiomyopathy is viral infection, especially coxsackievirus B3 (Table 1).

| Virus | Type | Patient positive (%) | |
		Myocarditis	Dilated cardiomyopathy
Picornavirus	*Coxackie A, B*	5-50%	5-15%
	Echovirus	?	?
	Hepatitis A	?	?
	Hepatitis C	*0-15%*	*0-10%*
Orthomyxovirus	Influenza A, B	?	?
Paramyxovirus	RSV, Mumpus	?	<1%
Rubivirus/Toga virus	Rubella virus	?	<1%
Rhabdo virus	Rabies virus	?	?
Arbovirus/Tahyna	Dengue, yellow fever virus	?	?
Retrovirus/Lenti	HIV	Variable	?
Herpes virus	*Varicella-zoster*	*1-2%*	*1-2%*
	Cytomegalovirus	*1-15%*	*1-10%*
	Epstein-Barr virus	*1-3%*	*1-3%*
	Human herpes virus 6	*0-5%*	*0-5%*
	herpes simplex virus	0-3%	?
Mastadenovirus	*Adenovirus*	*5-20%*	*10-12%*
Parvovirus	*Parvo B 19 virus*	*10-30%*	*10-25%*

Table 1. Virus-induced myocarditis or cardiomyopathy

Hoffmann et al also reported that IL-10 expression in human peripheral monocytes was strongly and persistently induced by coxsackievirus B3 infection in spite of only slight production of other pro-inflammatory cytokines such as TNF-α, IL-1 and IL-6 (20). It has been reported that the inhibition of natural killer (NK) cells results in increased virus titers in the heart through delayed virus clearance (21). IL-10 inhibits the production of IFN-γ in NK cells, which has been demonstrated in association with susceptibility to Trypanosoma cruzi-induced myocarditis (22-23). In addition, it has been shown that IL-10 is transcribed in the myocardium parallel with viral replication in the acute and chronic stages of experimental Coxsackievirus B3 viral myocarditis (24-25). These findings imply that an extreme elevation of serum levels of IL-10, rather than TNF-α, on admission may reflect subsequent myocardial inflammation, which leads to the future deterioration of the disease, through delayed clearance of the virus.

On the other hand, high levels of IL-10 may reflect a favorable long-term outcome in patients with acute myocarditis. Studies using experimental models have demonstrated a protective role of IL-10 in the development of acute myocarditis (26-27). This mechanism was explained by its suppressive effect against excessive and persistent immune response to viral infection or a subsequent autoimmune response leading to chronic myocardial injury. Cases with high level of IL-10 during acute phase may be not likely to develop to chronic myocarditis or cardiomyopathy. So far, almost studies with human myocarditis have been limited to a small number of patients. Further large number prospective studies are required to prove our idea.

In our previous study, the association of BNP with outcome was examined, also. Its levels in plasma were significantly increased in fulminant cases than in non-fulminant cases. However, we could not confirm its prognostic utility. In such cases, BNP may simply reflect the existence of circulatory failure alone.

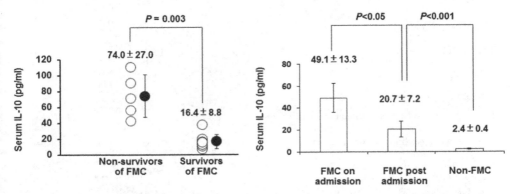

Serum levels of IL-10 were significantly increased in non-survivors than in survivors with fulminant myocarditis. IL-10 levels were significantly increased in not only patients with mechanical circulatory assist device on admission but also in those with it post admission, a few days after admission than in those without it throughout clinical course. IL: interleukin; FMC: fulminant myocarditis. (Nishii M, et al. J Am Coll Cardiol. 2004;44:1292-1297)

Fig. 1. Serum level of interleukin-10 in patients with acute myocarditis.

2.2.4 Cardiomyopathies

The HF is a major complication in cardiomyopathies such as dilated cardiomyopathy (DCM), hypertrophic cardiomyopathy (HCM), and restrictive cardiomyopathy (RCM). BNP must be a useful prognostic predictor for cardiomyopathies.

2.2.4.1 Dilated cardiomyopathy

Recently, we reported prognostic utility of BNP in clinically stable 83 outpatients with nonischemic DCM after decompensated HF (13). They were in a clinically stable status during at least 6 months after hospital discharge at relatively low BNP level, namely mean BNP level of about 200 pg/ml. This implied that pre-discharge BNP level may predict a post-discharge outcome in nonischemic DCM, as reported in general decompensated HF patients (12). Additionally, in this observation, the prognostic value of post-discharge BNP level was identified. Especially, among various predictors, levels at 6 months after hospital discharge showed the closest relation to the high risk of readmission for decompensated HF and mortality (Table 2). This association was explained by adverse cardiac remodeling. Persistently high levels of BNP during 6 months were related to poor improvement on cardiac remodeling (Figure 2).

Variable	Below vs. above median values			
	median level	HR	95% CI	P value
Univariate analysis				
Age	56	1.1895	0.7431-1.9246	0.47
Sex (Female)		1.0347	0.5886-2.0433	0.89
Hypertension		1.4902	0.8912-2.2819	0.18
Atrial fibrillation		1.2965	0.8885-2.0973	0.301
Ventricular tachycardia		1.2026	0.6132-2.1693	0.57
Beta-blocker use		1.6691	0.9056-2.5641	0.06
Diuretic use		1.3551	0.8086-2.1936	0.24
Echocardiographic parameters				
Left ventricular end-diastolic dimension at discharge	6.4 cm	0.8356	0.5189-1.3516	0.48
Left ventricular ejection fraction at discharge	30%	1.1629	0.7189-1.8729	0.54
Left atrial diastolic dimension at discharge	4.5 cm	1.3054	0.8106-2.1164	0.28
Left ventricular end-diastolic dimension at 6 months	6.0 cm	1.3866	0.8383-2.3598	0.22
Left ventricular ejection fraction at 6 months	36%	1.5019	0.9209-2.4641	0.11
Left atrial diastolic dimension at 6 months	4.25 cm	2.0003	1.2436-3.2233	0.0046
BNP measurements				
Plasma BNP level at discharge	180 pg/ml	1.2642	0.8051-1.9888	0.31
Plasma BNP level at 3 months	134 pg/ml	1.5097	0.9413-2.4212	0.09
Plasma BNP level at 6 months	174 pg/ml	2.2679	1.4336-3.5863	0.0005
Percentage change in BNP level between discharge and 3 months	-20.5%	1.4204	0.8863-2.2765	0.14
Percentage change in BNP level between discharge and 6 months	-11.5%	2.0127	1.2729-3.1757	0.0026
Multivariate analysis				
Plasma BNP level at 6 months	174 pg/ml	1.8427	1.1127-3.0426	0.0181
Percentage change in BNP level between discharge and 6 months	-11.5%	1.6538	0.9991-2.7214	0.051
Left atrial diastolic dimension at 6 months	4.25 cm	1.5678	0.9486-2.5904	0.0792

NYHA: New York Heart Association functional class; HR: hazard ratio; CI: confidence interval; BNP: B-type natriuretic peptide (Nishii M, et al. J Am Coll Cardiol. 2008;51:2329-2335)

Table 2. Univariate and multivariate Cox analyses of the incidence of death or readmission for heart failure.

2.2.4.2 Hypertrophic cardiomyopathy

Several reports have demonstrated that BNP levels reflect the severity of symptoms and HF in HCM (28-29). Additionally, high level of BNP has been related to cardiac events including silent myocardial ischemia (30), admission for HF, and mortality (31). On the other hand, our previous observation was unable to confirm these values, because even patients with high levels of BNP were in a clinically stable status. In HCM, BNP expression, however, is thought to occur as a response to not only hemodynamic changes resulting from diastolic dysfunction and obstruction but also histological changes such as myocardial fiber disarray, hypertrophy of myocytes, and fibrosis (32). Thus, even in clinically stable patients with HCM, extremely high levels may indicate a poor long-term outcome. Further studies are required to elucidate its prognostic value in HCM.

2.2.4.3 Restrictive cardiomyopathy

There is no report regarding prognostic value of BNP in RCM. However, when RCM had a further increase of LV end-diastolic pressure (LVEDP) or systolic dysfunction, BNP level would be more increased (7). BNP measurement may predict the occurrence of decompensated HF, although its value remains uncertain in RCM.

2.3 BNP-guided therapy

Efficiency of BNP-guided therapy on cardiomyopathies is not yet elucidated. However, BNP levels reflect therapeutic effect in patients with HF. Aggressive treatment with diuretics and vasodilators such as angiotensin-converting enzyme inhibitors (ACEIs) and angiotensin-II receptor antagonists reduce BNP level rapidly in conjunction with reduced intra-ventricular filling pressures. On the other hand, the effects of beta blockers on BNP concentrations are complex. Because adrenergic stimulation inhibits release of natriuretic peptides, beta blocking may initially increase BNP concentrations. By contrast, long-term use of beta blocker reduces BNP concentrations with the improvement in cardiac dysfunction. Thus, BNP measurement would help physicians to make clinical decisions to titrate pharmacological treatments.

BNP-guided therapy improves a treatment outcome in patients with HF. Two provocative pilot studies have prospectively assessed the utility of BNP to guide selection and intensity of pharmacotherapy. In one study, 69 symptomatic patients (NYHA class II to IV) with impaired systolic function defined as LVEF of <40% were randomly allocated to receive either standardised clinical assessment consist of symptoms and physical findings-guided therapy or N-terminal BNP-guided therapy (< 200 pmol/L) (33). During the follow up of at least 6 months, fewer patients had combined cardiovascular events (death, hospital admission, or heart failure decompensation) in the N-terminal BNP group than in the clinical group, which was associated with higher doses of ACEIs and diuretics. In a second multicenter randomised trial: The STARS-BNP Multicenter Study, 220 patients with symptomatic (NYHA class II to III) systolic HF defined as LVEF of <45% were randomized to medical treatments on either the basis of clinical findings from the physical examination and usual paraclinical and biological parameters or the basis of a decreasing BNP plasma levels of <100 pg/ml (34). After a mean follow-up of 15 months, significantly fewer patients had HF-related death in the BNP group than in the clinical group, which was in part associated with an increase in ACEIs and beta-blocker dosages.

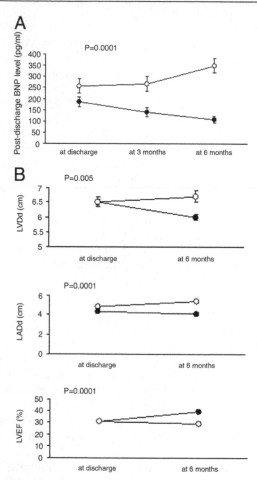

Fig. 2. Changes in B-type natriuretic peptide (BNP) levels and echocardiographic findings during a clinically compensated status in patients with dilated cardiomyopathy (Nishii M, et al. J Am Coll Cardiol. 2008;51:2329-2335)

Changes in BNP level at 3-month intervals after hospital discharge for decompensated heart failure (A) and in echocardiographic variables between discharge and 6 months (B). BNP levels were decreased during 6 months in event-free patients but not in readmitted patients, which was accompanied by the reduction of cardiac dimensions. Solid or open circles indicate BNP levels, echocardiographic dimensions (left ventricular end-diastolic dimension [LVDd]; left atrial diastolic dimension [LADd]), and left ventricular ejection fraction (LVEF) in event-free patients or patients readmitted for decompensated heart failure, respectively. Values are mean ± standard error of the mean. p values comparing changes in BNP and echocardiographic variables between readmitted patients and event-free patients are for repeated measures multivariate analysis of variance over 6 months.

On the other hand, it remained uncertain whether BNP guide is available for asymptomatic patients or not. We reported that in 83 outpatients with asymptomatic (NYHA class I to II) systolic HF defined as LVEF of <40%, BNP cutoff point of about 200 pg/ml at 6 months after the discharge for decompensated HF can identify patients at the high risk of readmission and sudden death (13) (Figure 3). Interestingly, Beta blocker use and its dosage were significantly lower in high risk patients [>200 vs. <200 pg/ml: 60 vs. 100%, P=0.001; 8 ± 5 vs. 16 ± 5 mg/day (carvedilol), P=0.0003; 64 ± 22 vs. 107 ± 40 mg/day (metoprolol), P=0.036; respectively]. The cutoff point might determine the requirement of initiation or titration of beta blockers. Even in asymptomatic HF setting, BNP-guided therapy may be also helpful.

2.4 The limitations on BNP-guided therapy
We have to consider the limitations on BNP-guided therapy, also. Recent multicenter trial (the randomized Trial of Intensified vs. Standard Medical Therapy in Elderly Patients with Congestive Heart Failure: TIME-CHF) could not identify the advantage of BNP-guided therapy over symptom-guided therapy in 499 elderly patients aged more than 60 years with symptomatic (NYHA class II or greater) systolic HF (LVEF of <45%) and prior hospitalization for decompensated HF (35). They were randomized to N-terminal BNP-guided HF therapy (levels of less than two times the upper limit of normal) and symptom-guided HF therapy (NYHA class of less than II). However, the improvements of outcomes including mortality, hospitalization, and quality of life were similar in both groups. Especially in patients aged more than 75 years, BNP-guided HF therapy did not improve outcome. In general, dosages of drugs such as ACEIs and beta-blockers are increased more in patients receiving BNP–guided therapy. Although persistence in intensifying medical therapy seems to be indispensable for better outcome in young and middle aged patients, it may be harmful to push dosages to the limits in elderly patients aged more than 75 years. Additionally, BNP-guided therapy may be disadvantageous in patients with low output syndrome resulting from severe systolic and diastolic dysfunctions. Because such cases require more ventricular load as a compensatory mechanism for congestive HF, rapid titration of ACEIs, beta blockers, and diuretics on the basis of BNP-guided HF therapy may lead to further deterioration of HF. Furthermore, edtablished cardiomyopathy with irreversible LV dilatation often shows persistently high level of BNP despite aggressive treatment for HF. A unified level of BNP-guided therapy would be unavailable for such cases. These emphasize the need of setting up individual BNP target level in accordance with cardiac conditions.

2.5 Individual target threshold of BNP
To set up individual target threshold of BNP for the risk reduction that were associated with cardiac dilatation and identify its prognostic utility, clinically stable 113 patients with systolic HF after decompensated HF represented by non-ischemic dilated cardiomyopathy were examined. Among these patients, 32 patients reached end-point composed of readmission for decompensated HF or death. Various variables were related to its combined event, including atrial fibrillation, low LVEF below the best cutoff value of 34%, cardiac dilatation (CD) indicated by left ventricular end-diastolic dimension×LAD/wall thickness/body surface area above the best cutoff value of 115 /m², high levels of BNP above the best cutoff value of 195 pg/ml. Furthermore, we found a significant positive correlation between BNP level and CD specific for event-free patients. The rage between 95% confidence interval on this specific linear regression line were closely associated with an incidence rate of readmission or death, also (Figure 4A, B). Thus, we defined this rage as individual target threshold of BNP.

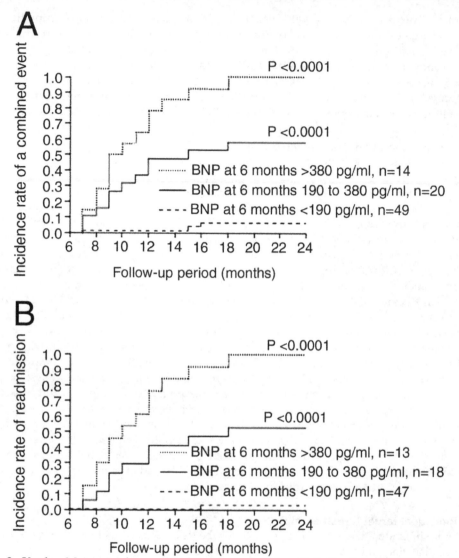

Fig. 3. Kaplan-Meier Analyses (Nishii M, et al. J Am Coll Cardiol. 2008;51:2329-2335) Kaplan-Meier curves showing the incidence rate of readmission for decompensated heart failure or sudden death (A) or of readmission alone (B) according to 6-month post-discharge B-type natriuretic peptide (BNP) ranges in outpatients with dilated cardiomyopathy. The risk of a combined event increased in a stepwise fashion across increasing ranges of 6-month post-discharge BNP, namely at <190 pg/ml, 190 to 380 pg/ml, and >380 pg/ml (Fig. 2A). Further, Kaplan-Meier curves for incidence of readmission alone (Fig. 2B) showed the same pattern. B-type natriuretic peptide ranges were <190 (the best cutoff level for predicting readmission or sudden death), 190 to 380, and >380 (its 2-fold level) pg/ml. p < 0.0001 (the log-rank test) versus a BNP range of <190 pg/ml.

Next, we examined its prognostic advantage over other variables. When adjusted to high-risk patients with advanced dilated cardiomyopathy, namely symptomatic non-ischemic systolic HF (LVEF below 34%) complicated by severe cardiac dilatation (CD above 115 /m²), this individual target threshold alone was associated with the incidence rate (Figure 5). Based on Laplace Law (pressure x radius/2 wall thickness), this threshold may reflect individual optimal wall stretch for clinical stabilization. The left atrium (LA) acts as a reservoir during LV overload (36), and elevated LV filling pressure results in LA overload as well as LV diastolic dysfunction (37). Thus, LA dimension reflects intra-ventricular pressure, in part.

A combined assessment of BNP level and echocardiographic dimensions may facilitate individual disease management. Among overall patients, those with BNP levels over or under its target threshold required titration or withdrawal, respectively of pharmocological therapy including diuretics or vosadilators to keep a balance between ventricular load and cardiac function. Additionally, cases refractory to such pharmacological optimization may be considered application of mechanical circulatory assist device implantation or subsequent surgical intervention including heart transplantation.

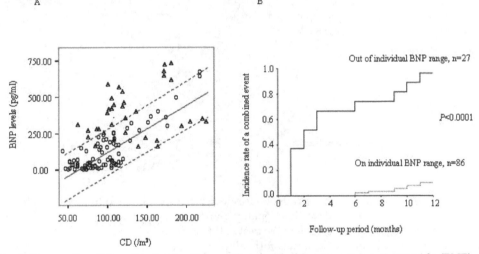

Fig. 4. Prognostic utility of individual target threshold of B-type natriuretic peptide (BNP) on readmission for decompensated heart failure or sudden death in patients with non-ischemic dilated cardiomyopathy

A: Individual target threshold of BNP. Event-free patients had a significantly positive correlation between BNP level and cardiac dilatation (CD) (r=0.88; P<0.0001), but event patients did not (r=0.26; P=0.421). BNP levels in event patients tended to be out of the range between dotted lines: 95% confidence interval (CI) on solid line: the linear regression line specific for event-free patients (BNP= -144.64 + 3.16×CD), namely individual target threshold of BNP. B: Kaplan-Meier curves showing the incidence rate of event according to individual target threshold of BNP. Out of this threshold was closely associated with an increase in event risk (the log-rank test: P<0.0001).

Open circles or triangles indicate even-free or event patients, respectively. CD was defined as left ventricular end-diastolic dimension×left atrial diastolic dimension/wall thickness/body surface area.

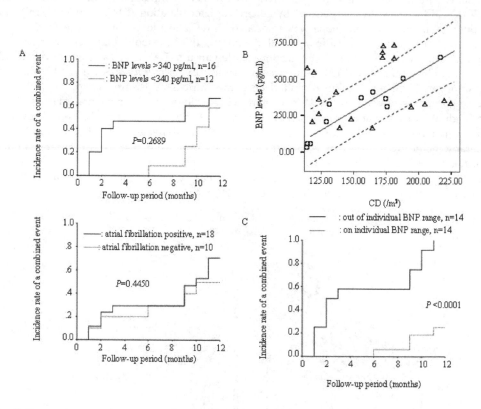

Fig. 5. Prognostic predictors on readmission for decompensated heart failure or death in patients with advanced dilated cardiomyopathy, namely symptomatic systolic heart failure (left ventricular ejection fraction below the best cutoff value of 34%) complicated by severe cardiac dilatation (CD) above the best cutoff value of 115 /m².

A: Kaplan-Meier curves showing the incidence rate of event according to levels of BNP above or below the best cutoff value of 340 pg/ml or atrial fibrillation. These variables had no significant association with an increase in event risk (the log-rank test; BNP levels: $P=0.2689$; atrial fibrillation: $P=0.4450$). B: Individual target threshold of BNP. Event-free patients had a significantly positive correlation between BNP level and CD ($r=0.91$; $P<0.0001$), independently of event patients ($r=0.10$; $P=0.71$). BNP levels in event patients tended to be out of individual target threshold of BNP between dotted lines: 95% confidence interval (CI) on solid line: the linear regression line specific for event-free patients C: Kaplan-Meier curves showing the incidence rate of event according to individual target threshold of BNP. Out of individual target threshold of BNP was significantly associated with an increase in event incidence (the log-rank test; $P<0.0001$).

Open circles or triangles indicate even-free or event patients. CD was defined as left ventricular end-diastolic dimension×left atrial diastolic dimension/wall thickness/body surface area.

The number of patients in our study is, however, relatively small, and our population was limited to only patients with non-ischemic dilated cardiomyopathy. Additional prospective multi-center studies including cases with ischemic heart disease would confirm our observation and extend it to various settings of systolic HF.

3. Conclusion

BNP measurement has facilitated the diagnosis of HF and decision of pharmacotherapy and improved outcome during the hospitalization and after the discharge for decompensated HF in cardiomyopathies, although BNP cutoff points for risk assessment are different on time course after decompensated HF and cardiac dysfunctions. On the other hand, availability of this BNP measurement was less especially in patients with advanced dilated cardiomyopathy as well as in elderly patients. However, individual target threshold of BNP for risk reduction related to cardiac dilatation exerted a strong prognostic power even in such advanced cases. This target threshold-guided therapy would facilitate individual disease management and thus contribute to further improvement of treatment outcome.

4. Acknowledgment

The authors thank Ms. Toshie Hashizume, Chiaki Notoya, and Kazumi Nakazato for their excellent technical assistance.

5. References

[1] Yoshimura, M.; Yasue, H.; Okumura, K.; Ogawa, H.; Jougasaki, M.; Mukoyama, M.; Nakao, K.; Imura, H. (1993). Different secretion pattern of atrial natriuretic peptide and brain natriuretic peptide in patients with congestive heart failure. *Circulation,* 87, 2, (Feb), pp. 464–469.

[2] Yasue, H.; Yoshimura, M and Sumida, H. (1994). Localization and mechanism of secretion of B-type natriuretic peptide in comparison with those of A-type natriuretic peptide in normal subjects and patients with heart failure. *Circulation,* 90, 1, (Jul), pp. 195–203.

[3] Brunner-La Rocca, HP.; Kaye, DM.; Woods, RL.; Hastings, J.; Esler, MD. (2001). Effects of intravenous brain natriuretic peptide on regional sympathetic activity in patients with chronic heart failure as compared with healthy control subjects. *J Am Coll Cardiol,* 37, 5, (Apr), pp. 1221–1227.

[4] Atarashi, K.; Mulrow, PJ.; Franco-Saenz, R. (1985). Effect of atrial peptides on aldosterone production. *J Clin Invest,* 76, 5, (Nov), pp. 1807–1811. .

[5] Maisel, AS.; Krishnaswamy, P.; Nowak, R.; McCord, J.; Hollander, JE.; Duc, P.; Omland, T.; Storrow, AB.; Abraham, WT.; Wu, AH.; Clopton, P.; Steg, PG.; Westheim, A.; Knudsen, CW.; Perez, A.; Kazanegra, R.; Herrmann, HC.; McCullough, PA. and Breathing Not Properly Multinational Study Investigators. (2002). Rapid measurement of B-type natriuretic peptide in the emergency diagnosis of heart failure. *N Engl J Med,* 347, 3, (Jul), pp. 161–167.

[6] Morrison LK, Harrison A, Krishnaswamy P, Kazanegra R, Clopton P, Maisel A. (2002). Utility of a rapid B-natriuretic peptide (BNP) assay in differentiating CHF from

lung disease in patients presenting with dyspnea. *J Am Coll Cardiol*, 39, 2, (Jan), pp. 202–209.

[7] Maisel, AS.; Koon, J.; Krishnaswamy, P.; Kazenegra, R.; Clopton, P.; Gardetto, N.; Morrisey, R.; Garcia, A.; Chiu, A.; De Maria, A. (2001). Utility of B-natriuretic peptide as a rapid, point-of-care test for screening patients undergoing echocardiography to determine left ventricular dysfunction. *Am Heart J*, 141, 3, (Mar), pp. 367–374.

[8] Yu CM, Sanderson JE, Shum IO, Chan S, Yeung LY, Hung YT, Cockram CS, Woo KS. (1996). Diastolic dysfunction and natriuretic peptides in systolic heart failure. Higher ANP and BNP levels are associated with the restrictive filling pattern. *Eur Heart J*, 17, 11, (Nov), pp. 1694-1702.

[9] Takeuchi, I.; Inomata, T.; Nishii, M.; Koitabashi, T.; Nakano, H.; Shinagawa, H.; Takehana, H.; Izumi, T. (2005). Clinical characteristics of heart disease patients with a good prognosis in spite of markedly increased plasma levels of type-B natriuretic peptide (BNP): anomalous behavior of plasma BNP in hypertrophic cardiomyopathy. Circ J, 69, 3, (Mar), pp. 277-282.

[10] Leya, FS.; Arab, D.; Joyal, D.; Shioura, KM.; Lewis, BE.; Steen, LH.; Cho, L. (2005). The efficacy of brain natriuretic peptide levels in differentiating constrictive pericarditis from restrictive cardiomyopathy. *J Am Coll Cardiol*. 45, 11, (Jun), pp. 1900-1902.

[11] Fonarow, GC.; Peacock, WF.; Phillips, CO.; Givertz, MM.; Lopatin, M.; ADHERE Scientific Advisory Committee and Investigators. (2007). Admission B-type natriuretic peptide levels and in-hospital mortality in acute decompensated heart failure. *J Am Coll Cardiol*, 49, 19, (May), pp. 1943-1950.

[12] Logeart, D.; Thabut, G.; Jourdain, P.; Chavelas, C.; Beyne, P.; Beauvais, F.; Bouvier, E.; Solal, AC. (2004). Predischarge B-type natriuretic peptide assay for identifying patients at high risk of re-admission after decompensated heart failure. *J Am Coll Cardiol*, 43, 4, (Feb), pp. 635-641.

[13] Nishii, M.; Inomata, T.; Takehana, H.; Naruke, T.; Yanagisawa, T.; Moriguchi, M.; Takeda, S.; Izumi, T. (2008). Prognostic utility of B-type natriuretic peptide assessment in stable low-risk outpatients with nonischemic cardiomyopathy after decompensated heart failure. *J Am Coll Cardiol*, 51, 24, (Jun), pp. 2329-2335.

[14] Richards, AM.; Nicholls, MG.; Yandle, TG.; Frampton, C.; Espiner, EA.; Turner, JG.; Buttimore, RC.; Lainchbury, JG.; Elliott, JM.; Ikram, H.; Crozier, IG.; Smyth, DW. (1998). Plasma N-terminal pro-brain natriuretic peptide and adrenomedullin: new neurohormonal predictors of left ventricular function and prognosis after myocardial infarction. *Circulation*, 97, 19, (May), pp. 1921-1929.

[15] de Lemos, JA.; Morrow, DA.; Bentley, JH.; Omland, T.; Sabatine, MS.; McCabe, CH.; Hall, C.; Cannon, CP.; Braunwald, E. (2001). The prognostic value of B-type natriuretic peptide in patients with acute coronary syndromes. *N Engl J Med*, 345, 14 (Oct), pp. 1014-1021.

[16] Lieberman, EB.; Hutchins, GM.; Herskowitz, A.; Rose, NR.; Baughman, KL. (1991). Clinicopathologic description of myocarditis. *J Am Coll Cardiol*, 18, 7, (Dec), pp. 1617-1626.

[17] McCarthy, RE 3 rd.; Boehmer, JP.; Hruban, RH.; Hutchins, GM.; Kasper, EK.; Hare, JM.; Baughman, KL. (2000). Long-term outcome of fulminant myocarditis as compared with acute (nonfulminant) myocarditis. *New Engl J Med*, 342, 10, (Mar), pp. 690-695.

[18] Woodruff, JF. Viral myocarditis: a review. (1980). Am J Pathol, 101, 2, (Nov), pp. 425-484.

[19] Nishii, M.; Inomata, T.; Takehana, H.; Takeuchi, I.; Nakano, H.; Koitabashi, T.; Nakahata, J.; Aoyama, N.; Izumi, T. (2004). Serum levels of interleukin-10 on admission as a prognostic predictor of human fulminant myocarditis. *Am J Coll Cardiol*, 44, 6, (Sep),pp. 1292-1297.

[20] Hofmann, P.; Schmidtke, M.; Stelzer, A.; Gemsa, D. (2001). Suppression of Proinflammatory cytokines and induction of IL-10 in human monocytes after coxsackievirus B3 infection. *J Med Virol*, 64, 4, (Aug), pp. 487-98.

[21] Godeny, EK.; Gauntt, CJ. (1987). Murine natural killer cells limit coxsackievirus B3 replication. *J Immunol*, 139, 3, (Aug), pp. 913-918.

[22] Reed, SG.; Brownell, CE.; Russo, DM.; Siva, JS.; Grabstein, KH.; Morrissey, PJ. (1994). IL-10 mediates susceptibility to Trypanosoma cruzi infection. *J Immunol*, 153, 7, (Oct), pp. 3135-3140.

[23] Silva, JS.; Aliberti, JC.; Martin, GA.; Souza, M.; Souto, JT.; Padua, MA. (1998). The role of IL-12 in experimental Trypanosoma cruzi infection. *Braz J Med Biol Res*, 31, 1, (Jan), pp. 111-115.

[24] Gluck, B.; Schmidtke, M.; Merkle, I.; Stelzner, A.; Gemsa, D. (2001). Persistent expression of cytokines in the chronic stage of CVB3-induced myocarditis in NMRI mice. *J Moll Cell Cardiol*, 33, 9, (Sep), pp. 1615-1626.

[25] Schmidtke, M.; Gluck, B.; Merkle, I.; Hoffmann, P.; Stelzner, A.; Gemsa, D. (2000). Cytokine profiles in heart, spleen, and thymus during the acute stage of experimental coxsackievirus B3-induced chronic myocarditis. *J Med Virol*, 61, 4, (Aug), pp. 518-526.

[26] Watanabe, K.; Nakazawa, M.; Fuse, K.; Hanawa, H.; Kodama, M.; Aizawa, Y.; Ohnuki, T.; Gejyo, F.; Maruyama, H.; Miyazaki, J. (2001). Protection against autoimmune myocarditis by gene transfer of interleukin-10 by electroporation. *Circulation*, 104, 10, (Sep), pp. 1098-1100.

[27] Nishio, R.; Matsumori, A.; Shioi, T.; Ishida, H.; Sasayama, S. (1999). Treatment of Experimental Viral Myocarditis With Interleukin-10. *Circulation*, 100, 10, (Sep), pp. 1102-1108.

[28] Maron, BJ.; Tholakanahalli, VN.; Zenovich, AG.; Casey, SA.; Duprez, D.; Aeppli, DM.; Cohn, JN. (2004). Usefulness of B-type natriuretic peptide assay in the assessment of symptomatic state in hypertrophic cardiomyopathy. *Circulation*, 109, 8, (Mar), pp. 984-989.

[29] Arteaga, E.; Araujo, AQ.; Buck, P.; Ianni, BM.; Rabello, R.; Mady, C. (2005). Plasma amino-terminal pro-B-type natriuretic peptide quantification in hypertrophic cardiomyopathy. *Am Heart J*, 150, 6, (Dec), pp. 1228-1232.

[30] Nakamura, T.; Sakamoto, K.; Yamano, T.; Kikkawa, M.; Zen, K.; Hikosaka, T.; Kubota, T.; Azuma, A.; Nishimura, T. (2002). Increased plasma brain natriuretic peptide level as a guide for silent myocardial ischemia in patients with non-obstructive hypertrophic cardiomyopathy. *J Am Coll Cardiol*, 39, 10, (May), pp. 1657-1663.

[31] Kubo, T.; Kitaoka, H.; Okawa, M.; Yamanaka, S.; Hirota, T.; Baba, Y.; Hayato, K.; Yamasaki, N.; Matsumura, Y.; Yasuda, N.; Sugiura, T.; Doi, YL. (2011). Combined measurements of cardiac troponin I and brain natriuretic Peptide are useful for predicting adverse outcomes in hypertrophic cardiomyopathy. *Circ J*, 75, 4, (Mar), pp. 919-926.

[32] Hasegawa, K.; Fujiwara, H.; Doyama, K.; Miyamae, M.; Fujiwara, T.; Suga, S.; Mukoyama, M.; Nakao, K.; Imura, H.; Sasayama, S. (1993). Ventricular expression of brain natriuretic peptide in hypertrophic cardiomyopathy. *Circulation*, 88, 2, (Aug), pp. 372-380.

[33] Troughton, RW.; Frampton, CM,; Yandle, TG.; Espiner, EA.; Nicholls, MG.; Richards, AM. (2000). Treatment of heart failure guided by plasma aminoterminal brain natriuretic peptide (N-BNP) concentrations. *Lancet*, 355, 9210, (Apr), pp. 1126-1130.

[34] Jourdain, P.; Jondeau, G.; Funck, F.; Gueffet, P.; Le Helloco, A.; Donal, E.; Aupetit, JF.; Aumont, MC.; Galinier, M.; Eicher, JC.; Cohen-Solal, A.; Juillière, Y. (2007). Plasma brain natriuretic peptide-guided therapy to improve outcome in heart failure: the STARS-BNP Multicenter Study. *J Am Coll Cardiol*, 49, 16, (Apr), pp. 1733-1739.

[35] Pfisterer, M.; Buser, P.; Rickli, H.; Gutmann, M.; Erne, P.; Rickenbacher, P.; Vuillomenet, A.; Jeker, U.; Dubach, P.; Beer, H.; Yoon, SI.; Suter, T.; Osterhues, HH.; Schieber, MM.; Hilti, P.; Schindler, R.; Brunner-La Rocca, HP.; TIME-CHF Investigators. (2009). BNP-guided vs. symptom-guided heart failure therapy: the Trial of Intensified vs. Standard Medical Therapy in Elderly Patients with Congestive Heart Failure (TIME-CHF) randomized trial. *JAMA*, 301, 4, (Jan), pp. 383–392.

[36] Hoit, BD.; Shao, Y.; Gabel, M.; Walsh, RA. (1994). In vivo assessment of left atrial contractile performance in normal and pathological conditions using a time-varying elastance model. *Circulation*, 89, 4, (Apr), pp. 1829-1838.

[37] Dernellis, JM.; Stefanadis, CI.; Zacharoulis, AA.; Toutouzas, PK. (1998). Left atrial mechanical adaptation to long-standing hemodynamic loads based on pressure-volume relations. *Am J Cardiol*, 81, 9, (May), pp. 1138-1143.

5

Management of Hypertrophic Obstructive Cardiomyopathy with a Focus on Alcohol Septal Ablation

Josef Veselka
Department of Cardiology, 2nd Medical School, Charles University,
University Hospital Motol, Prague
Czech Republic

1. Introduction

Hypertrophic cardiomyopathy (HCM) is a complex cardiac disease with unique pathophysiological characteristics and a great diversity of morphological, functional, and clinical features. HCM is defined as primary myocardial hypertrophy in the absence of aortic valve disease or significant hypertension (Elliott, 2008)

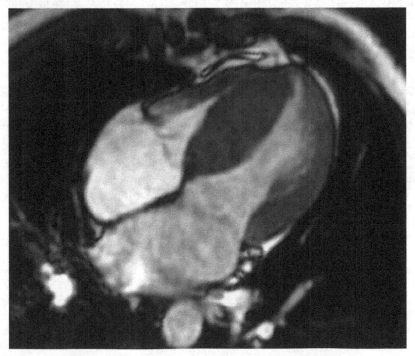

Fig. 1. Magnetic resonance imaging; hypertrophic left and right ventricle.

Several observations suggest that the prevalence of HCM is globally 1 in 500 (Maron, 1994). The condition therefore seems to be a common genetic malformation of the heart. The clinical course varies markedly. Some patients remain asymptomatic throughout their whole lives, some have severe symptomatology of heart failure or angina pectoris, while others die suddenly even in the absence of previous symptoms. The annual mortality rate varies in different studies. In unselected populations, it has been reported to be about 1% (Elliott, 2008). These observations suggest that a substantial proportion of patients with HCM has a more favourable course than previously believed. Two thirds of patients with HCM display evidence of obstruction in the left ventricular outflow tract (hypertrophic obstructive cardiomyopathy, HOCM), that is negatively associated with prognosis of the patients.

During the last decade, technological developments in non-surgical treatment have provided new therapeutic options for patients with this disease. Recent changes have also generated considerable questions about the optimal management of HOCM and the role of percutaneous alcohol septal ablation (ASA) (Veselka, 2007).

With respect to various clinical courses, it seems to be impossible to define precise guidelines for management. As in many diseases, it is often necessary to individualise therapy.

2. Drug therapy of patients with hypertrophic obstructive cardiomyopathy

Drug therapy is used as the initial measure for controlling cardiac symptoms that has resulted in functional limitation. Beta-blockers and verapamil have traditionally been administered on an empirical basis, relying on the patient´s subjective perception of benefit. Drug selection is based on preferences of individual physicians. Most favour beta-blockers over verapamil for use in initial treatment, although it is not of critical importance which drug is used first.

There is no evidence that beta-blockers or verapamil protect patients with HOCM from sudden death. On the other hand, they are able to relieve symptoms in the majority of patients. Whether these drugs should be used prophylactically to delay disease progression and improve prognosis in asymptomatic patients has been a subject of debate for many years. The effectiveness of a prophylactic treatment has not been tested prospectively because study populations are small and traditional endpoints are infrequent (death, clinical deterioration). Accordingly, we reserve medical therapy only for symptomatic patients.

3. Surgery to relieve the left ventricular obstruction

The group of patients who have both a large outflow gradient and severe symptoms and also do not respond to medical treatment are the best candidates for surgery. Based on outstanding experience of several surgical centres worldwide, myectomy has become the primary therapeutic option for patients with severe symptoms and marked functional disability (McCully, 1996). Surgical reduction of the outflow gradient is achieved by removing a small amount of muscle (5 to 10 g) from the basal septum. Recently, some surgeons have performed more extended myectomies and reconstruction of the subvalvular mitral apparatus. In these cases, the septal myectomy deeply extends into the left ventricular cavity. Subsequently, both papillary muscles are mobilised and all hypertrophied muscular trabeculae are also resected. Mitral valve replacement has also been used as an alternative therapy in selected patients, but the role of this operation remains unsettled.

Surgery substantially reduces the basal outflow gradient in more than 90% of patients and provides large improvements in objective measures of symptoms and functional status.

However, the procedure requires extracorporeal circulation and great surgical experience. Mortality rates less than 2% are achieved only in heart centres with extensive surgical experience and numerous performed procedures. The effect of surgery on survival is not known. Accordingly, surgery is not performed in asymptomatic or mildly symptomatic patients.

4. Cardiac pacing to relieve the left ventricular obstruction

The role of cardiac pacing in reducing the left ventricular outflow gradient in HOCM was first reported more than 40 years ago (Gilgenkrantz, 1968). At the same time, it had been noticed that patients who developed left bundle branch block after septal myectomy had a better functional outcome. Sporadic reports over the years have culminated in the interest of cardiac pacing in the 1990s´.

In the early 1990s, several observational studies reported that dual-chamber pacing with shortened A-V delay was associated with both substantial decrease in the outflow gradient and symptomatic improvement of patients unresponsive to drug treatment. However, the mechanisms by which pacing might reduce outflow gradient was not understood. Later, three more carefully controlled and randomised studies found the effects of cardiac pacing to be less favourable (Linde, 1999; Maron, 1999; Nishimura, 1997). These studies were randomised, double-blind and crossover. Subjective symptomatic improvement was reported with similar frequency by patients after three months pacing and after the same period without pacing. Objective measurements of exercise capacity (for example maximal oxygen consumption) with and without pacing did not differ significantly. These findings suggested that a placebo effect might play an important role in the symptomatic improvement reported by the paced patients. Currently, cardiac pacing cannot be regarded as a primary treatment for patients with HOCM, although a modest reduction in outflow gradient is achieved in a number of paced patients. Probably a small subset of patients could profit from pacing, but this effect is inconsistent and usually only modest. Therefore, further randomized, controlled trials should be undertaken to resolve the uncertainties surrounding the utility and efficacy of cardiac pacing in patients with HOCM.

5. Alcohol septal ablation to relieve the left ventricular obstruction

The idea of inducing a septal infarction by catheter techniques was suggested by the observation that myocardial function of selected areas of the left ventricle can be suppressed by balloon occlusion of the supplying artery during angioplasty. The outflow pressure gradient in HOCM decreased significantly when the first septal artery was temporarily occluded by an angioplasty balloon catheter (Sigwart, 1982). This concept was also supported by observations that the outflow pressure gradient decreased after anterior myocardial infarction in HOCM patients.

Sigwart published his experience with "non-surgical myocardial reduction" of three patients with HOCM in 1995 (Sigwart, 1995). However, at the same time, other centres in Germany also started with the same interventional procedure (Kuhn, 2010). Since then, several modifications of the original technique have been described. The majority of authors prefer an echocardiography-guided anatomical approach for identifying the target septal branch (Veselka, 2007), where the target septal branch is detected using myocardial contrast echocardiography (MCE). Estimation of the size of the septal vascular territory with MCE is accurate and safe. Using MCE, it is possible to delineate the perfusion bed of the septal perforators and predict the infarct size that follows the alcohol injection.

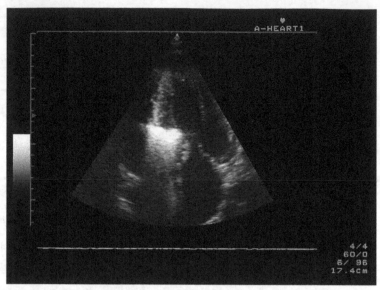

Fig. 2. Transthoracic echocardiography, apical 4-chamber view with optimal opacification of the basal interventricular septum by echocontrast medium.

Recently, we have proposed the use of real-time myocardial contrast echocardiography with very low mechanical index that allows better delineation of the target area than conventional contrast echocardiography (Veselka, 2009).

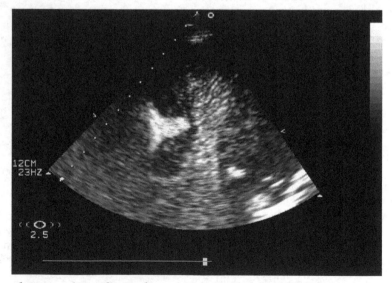

Fig. 3. Transthoracic echocardiography, apical 4-chamber view with real time myocardial contrast echocardiography utilizing power modulation and intracoronary injection of small amount of echocontrast agent.

There is a significant correlation between MCE septal area and reduction of ouflow gradient. In general, a higher biomarker level (extent of necrosis) was detected with larger sections of the infarcted septum. However, since alcohol injection is directed mainly to the portion of the septum causing the obstruction, many patients have a small defect with a large reduction of outflow gradient. Additionally, it has been found that MCE in 5 to 10% of cases shows contrast within myocardium away from the septal target area, indicating threatening misplacement of the myocardial necrosis. Accordingly, necrotisation of myocardium distant from the septal target area as a source of potentially fatal complications can be avoided by this approach. The introduction of echocardiographic guidance of ASA led to an improvement in haemodynamic results, despite a decrease in the infarcted septal area estimated by the maximal creatine kinase rise.

5.1 Indication
Accepted patient selection criteria for ASA were as follows: (1) anatomical findings of marked septal hypertrophy that projects from the LVOT; (2) dynamic obstruction of LVOT; (3) unresponsiveness to the medical therapy. There were no sufficient data available to confirm exact haemodynamic (pressure gradient > 50 mmHg), anatomical (septum thickness > 18 mm) or clinical (dyspnoea with NYHA class III or IV) criteria that resulted in a certain relaxation of indications in clinical practice. Patients with moderate symptoms were treated if they had high gradients and additional findings, such as recurrent exercise-induced syncope, markedly abnormal blood pressure response at exercise, paroxysmal atrial fibrillation or extremely high pressure gradient after provocative manoeuvres (Valsalva manoeuvre or use of nitrates). It is a very important question in clinical practice whether the increased risk of sudden cardiac death associated with LVOT obstruction justifies the use of ASA in slightly symptomatic or completely asymptomatic patients. At present, there are no sufficient data to answer this question. However, a relatively low risk of sudden death in asymptomatic patients with obstruction and none of the recognised risk factors for sudden death (1.ventricular tachycardia, 2. abnormal exercise blood pressure response, 3. family history of premature death, 4. unexplained syncope, 5. severe left ventricular hypertrophy in any myocardial segment > 30 mm) suggests that aggressive interventions are unjustified in this group. The situation in asymptomatic patients with obstruction and additional risk factors is less clear. The approach must be individualised. It seems to be reasonable to implant an AV-sequential implantable cardioverter-defibrillator (ICD) to try atrio-ventricular sequential pacing to reduce obstruction for 6 months, and then to perform ASA if needed. Nevertheless, ASA as the primary treatment is still unjustified in this group of patients, given potential mortality and morbidity associated with this procedure. Patient preference should, of course, be considered in such discussion and surgical myectomy should be mentioned as the gold standard in most western countries.

5.2 Alcohol septal ablation procedure
We usually recommend the following course of ASA procedure. A temporary pacemaker is placed in the apex of the right ventricle in everyone except patients who already have a permanent dual-chamber pacemaker in place. However, fluctuation of the pacing threshold has to be anticipated if the lead is directed towards the septum, i.e., with the tip in proximity to the ablation lesion. A multipurpose catheter is advanced through the aortic valve into the

apex of the left ventricle and intraventricular gradient is measured by a pull-back technique. A 6 or 7F guiding catheter is then engaged into the ostium of the left coronary artery. Initial angiography is performed to localise the origin of septal arteries. Over-the-wire balloon catheter is introduced over a coronary wire into one of the major and proximal septal perforators and inflated. Contrast medium is injected through the central balloon lumen to delineate the area supplied by the septal branch and to ensure that balloon inflation prevents spillage into the left anterior descending artery. Contrast myocardial echocardiography is performed to delineate the area to be infarcted (Figures 1 and 2) and to exclude contrast (and subsequently alcohol) deposition in remote myocardial regions like the left ventricular posterior wall or papillary muscles. The optimal septal branch is identified by opacification of the area in the basal septum that is adjacent to the zone of maximal acceleration of the outflow jet and includes the point of coaptation between the septum and anterior mitral leaflet. Usually, the target septal branch originates from the proximal segment of the left anterior descending artery. However, in exceptional cases, it originates from diagonal or intermediate branches of the left coronary artery. Depending on the septal artery size and septal thickness, 1 to 2 ml of absolute ethanol are very slowly (2 to 3 minutes) instilled through the lumen of the inflated balloon catheter and left in place for 5 minutes. After balloon deflation and removal, angiography is done to confirm the patency of the left anterior descending artery and occlusion of the target septal branch. Measurement of intraventricular gradient is usually performed by a multipurpose catheter and guiding catheter and/or Doppler echocardiography. The gradient should decrease at least to one half.

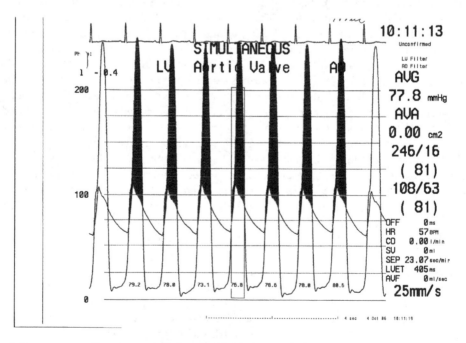

Fig. 4. Pressure gradient between left ventricle and aorta before ASA.

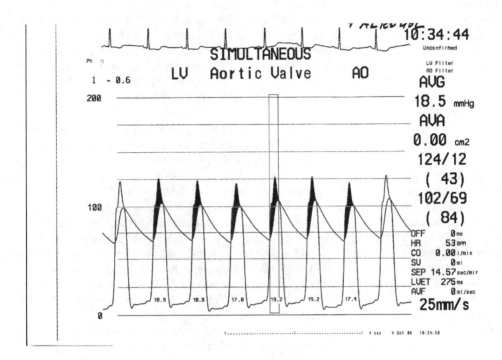

Fig. 5. Hemodynamic finding after ASA with nearly elimination of pressure gradient after procedure.

A temporary pacemaker is sutured in place. The patient is observed in the coronary care unit for at least 48 hours. If there is no high-degree atrioventricular block, the pacemaker lead is then removed.

5.3 Complications

In-hospital death, the most significant complication of ASA, is rare. Nevertheless, it ranges in the literature from 1 to 4%. However, some observations suggest that in skilled hands, the mortality rate is close to zero.

Historically, the incidence of complete heart block following ASA has ranged from 0 to 40% with a mean value of 8 to 18% (Veselka, 2007). However, the original technique of ASA has undergone several modifications and lower occurrence of post-procedural complete heart block has been reported (Veselka, 2010). The most important trend in the continuously developing ASA technique involves the lowering of the alcohol dose (1 to 2 ml) injected in very small fractions (0.1 to 0.3 ml) (Veselka, 2005). Subsequent small infarctions are sufficient in reducing obstruction to a similar extent as larger infarctions induced by a higher dose of alcohol. Moreover, it seems to be likely that a low dose of alcohol is associated with lower incidence of major post-procedural conduction disturbances and improved prognosis (Kuhn, 2008).

The selection of appropriate patients for this procedure appears to be as important as the procedural ASA technique itself. Only highly symptomatic patients without the left bundle branch block should be treated by ASA because of high incidence of right bundle branch block following ASA. Unfortunately, the resulting complete heart block can occur with no previous symptoms within hours or days after the procedure. Therefore, based on our clinical experience, patients after uncomplicated ASA should be observed in the coronary care unit for at least 2 or 3 days and consequent telemetric monitoring should be considered for at least 1 week.

To improve the risk stratification of complete heart block occurrence, Faber et al. proposed a scoring system based on baseline ECG, heart rate profile, severity of obstruction, peri-interventional enzyme kinetics, and peri-interventional conduction problems that might discriminate patients with a high risk for permanent pacemaker dependency from those with a stable atrioventricular conduction after ASA (Faber, 2007).

Sustained ventricular tachycardia has been rarely reported following ASA and only few reports have described it as an early post-procedural complication (Veselka, 2010). There is the hypothesis that the early post-procedural period can be compared to the same period after acute myocardial infarction, and the development of sustained ventricular arrhythmias after the ASA is not as rare as was thought before. It seems to be likely that a lower dose of alcohol with the minimising of the resulting necrosis (scar) is unable to entirely eliminate either occurrence of ventricular arrhythmias that are dependent on disorganised cellular architecture of myocardium or serious conduction abnormalities.

Still, some uncertainty persists regarding the ICD indication for the prevention of sudden death in patients with post-procedural sustained ventricular arrhythmias, and no data are available regarding their predictive power. Nevertheless, based on both our clinical experience (and lack of scientific evidence), we do not consider early post-procedural ventricular arrhythmias to be a sufficient justification per se for an ICD implantation.

A serious complication of ASA is a leakage of ethanol from the target septal branch into the left anterior descending artery. This potentially fatal complication is avoided by the use of a slightly over-sized angioplasty balloon catheter and a very careful septal branch angiography that precedes alcohol ablation. Additionally, the slow administration of alcohol per fractions and septal branch occlusion for 5 minutes after the last alcohol injection ensure the safe course of the procedure.

Theoretically, the potential risk of ventricular septal rupture following ASA should be considered. Surprisingly, this serious complication is probably very rare, although it is possible that it is underreported in the literature.

5.4 Results

ASA has not been subjected to many randomised clinical trials. However, observational data from European and US centres over a 16-year follow-up are consistent, attributing a number of favourable effects to ASA that generally parallel that of surgery, including gradual and progressive reduction in outflow gradient over 3 to 12 months and alleviation of symptoms.

The most important finding after ASA is an impressive symptomatic improvement during both short- and long-term follow-up that is consistently reported by all groups dealing with

ASA. The mean functional class improved very significantly from NYHA 2.5-3 to 1.2-1.6. Similarly, objective measurements showed an increase in exercise capacity and peak oxygen consumption.

During ASA, an acute LVOT gradient reduction is followed by a significant LVOT gradient increase during the early post-procedural period and a continuous LVOT gradient decrease during the follow-up. The rapid post-procedural LVOT gradient decrease is probably associated mainly with stunning, myocardial necrosis and the change in the left ventricular ejection dynamics. The later pressure gradient decrease is caused by scarring and thinning of the basal septum, resulting in left ventricular remodelling (Veselka, 2004).

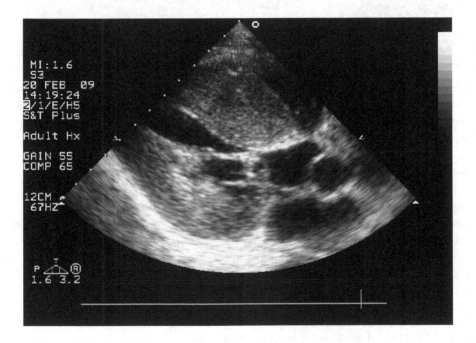

Fig. 6. Transthoracic echocardiography, parasternal long axis view with impressive finding of subaortic obstruction.

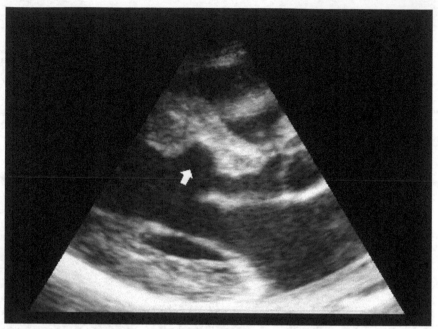

Fig. 7. Transthoracic echocardiography, parasternal long axis view with thinning of the basal interventricular septum (arrow) three months following ASA.

This haemodynamic course characterised by "down-up-down" changes in pressure gradient occurs in the majority of patients and is called the "biphasic" response. In most trials, the resting LVOT pressure gradient is reduced from 60 to 70 mmHg at baseline to 10 to 20 mmHg at mid- or long-term follow-up.

6. Conclusion

At present, there is not a single therapy that should be applied to all patients with severely symptomatic HOCM unresponsive to medical management. There are benefits and disadvantages of both surgical myectomy and ASA. Septal myectomy requires specialised tertiary referral centres and is a more complex procedure than ASA. Furthermore, there is no cardio-thoracic surgical centre in our country that would be able to perform this procedure routinely. On the other hand, there are no sufficient data concerning the long-term follow-up of patients after ASA.

Further investigation is required to be able to identify the best responders for cardiac pacing, ASA and surgical myectomy and compare the results for the available methods. Mainly, a randomised study comparing myectomy and ASA would be needed. However, low incidence of end points would require extremely high number of participants and, therefore, such a study will probably not be performed.

Currently, a decision concerning the best therapy of patients with HOCM must be individualised to each patient depending on their wishes and expectations, way of life, age and haemodynamics. Centres of excellence are able to perform both ASA and myectomy very safely and effectively. Therefore, choice of the final therapy should be tailored for the individual patient treated in a particular centre.

7. References

Elliott P, Anderson B, Arbustini E, et al. *Classification of the cardiomyopathies: a position statement from the European Society of Cardiology working group on myocardial and pericardial diseases.* Eur Heart J 2008;29:270-6.

Faber L, Welge D, Fassbender D, Schmidt HK, Horstkotte D, Seggewiss H. *One-year follow-up of percutaneous septal ablation for symptomatic hypertrophic obstructive cardiomyopathy in 312 patients: predictors of hemodynamic and clinical response.* Clin Res Cardiol 2007;96:864-873.

Gilgenkrantz J, Cherrier F, Petitier H, Dodinot B, Houplon M, Legoux J. *Cardiomyopathie obstructive du ventricle gauche avec block auriculo-ventriculaire complet. Considerations therapeutiques.* Arch Mal Coeur 1968;61:439-53.

Kuhn H, Lawrenz T, Lieder F, Leuner C, Strunk-Mueller C, Obergassel L, Bartelsmeier M, Stellbrink C. *Survival after transcoronary ablation of septal hypertrophy in hypertrophic obstructive cardiomyopathy (TASH): a 10year experience.* Clin Res Cardiol 2008;97:243-34.

Kuhn HJ. *The history of alcohol septal ablation.* Cardiovasc Revasc Med 2010;11:260-261.

Linde C, Gadler F, Kappenberger L, et al. *Placebo effect of pacemaker implantation in obstructive hypertrophic cardiomyopathy.* Am J Cardiol 1999;83:903-7.

Maron BJ, Gardin JM, Flack JM, Kurosaki TT, Bild TE. *Prevalence of hypertrophic cardiomyopathy in general population of young adults: echocardiographic analysis of 4111 subjects in the CARDIA study.* Circulation 1995;92:785-9.

Maron BJ, Nishimura RA, McKenna WJ, et al. *Assessment of permanent dual-chamber pacing as a treatment for drug-refractory symptomatic patients with obstructive hypertrophic cardiomyopathy. A randomized, double-blind, crossover study (M-PATHY).* Circulation 1999;99:2927-2933.

McCully RB, Nishimura RA, Tajik AJ, et al. *Extent of clinical improvement after surgical treatment of hypertrophic obstructive cardiomyopathy.* Circulation 1996;94:467-71.

Nishimura RA, Trusty J, Hayes DL, et al. *Dual-chamber pacing for hypertrophic cardiomyopathy: a randomised, double-blind, crossover trial.* J Am Coll Cardiol 1997;435-441.

Sigwart U, Grbie M, Essinger A, Rivier JL. *L´effet aigu d´une occlusion coronarienne par ballonet de la dilatation transluminale.* Schweiz Med Wochenschr 1982;45:1631.

Sigwart U. *Non-surgical myocardial reduction of hypertrophic obstructive cardiomyopathy.* Lancet 1995;346:211-4.

Veselka J, Duchoňová R, Procházková Š, Homolová I, Páleníčková J, Zemánek D, Pernišová Z, Tesař D. *The biphasic course of changes of left ventricular outflow gradient after alcohol septal ablation for hypertrophic obstructive cardiomyopathy.* Kardiol Pol 2004;60:133-5.

Veselka J, Duchoňová R, Procházková Š, Páleníčková J, Sorajja P, Tesař D. *Effects of varying ethanol dosing in percutaneous septal ablation for obstructive hypertrophic cardiomyopathy on early hemodynamic ganges.* Am J Cardiol 2005;95:675-8.

Veselka J. *Alcohol septal ablation for hypertrophic obstructive cardiomyopathy: a review of the literature.* Med Sci Monit 2007;13:RA62-8.

Veselka J, Zemánek D, Fiedler J, Šváb P. *Real-time myocardial contrast echocardiography for echo-guided alcohol septal ablation*. Arch Med Sci 2009;5:271-272.

Veselka J, Zemánek D, Tomašov P, Homolová S, Adlová R, Tesař D. *Complications of low-dose echo-guided alcohol septal ablation*. Catheter Cardiovasc Interv 2010;75:546-550.

6

Hypertrophic Cardiomyopathy in Infants and Children

Luis E. Alday and Eduardo Moreyra

Divisions of Cardiology, Hospital Aeronáutico and Sanatorio Allende, Córdoba
Argentina

1. Introduction

The definition and classification of the cardiomyopathies has been traditionally a complex and quite variable subject. In 2006, the American Heart Association issued a scientific statement elaborated by a task force of experts that contemplated the important development of molecular genetics in recent years, to explain the etiology of the diseases of cardiac muscle, or cardiomyopathies, previously considered idiopathic (B.J. Maron et al., 2006a). The document stated that "Cardiomyopathies are an heterogeneous group of myocardial diseases associated with mechanical and/or electrical dysfunction that usually, but not always, exhibit inappropriate ventricular hypertrophy or dilation, and are originated by a variety of causes, frequently genetic. Cardiomyopathies involve just the heart or are part of systemic disorders that often lead to cardiovascular death or heart failure related disability". Myocardial damage secondary to coronary atherosclerosis, heart valve disease, congenital heart disease, and systemic hypertension, is excluded from this definition. Primary or metastatic cardiac tumors and diseases primarily affecting the endocardium with minimal or absent myocardial damage neither are included. The document also discourages the use of the classical terminologies hypertrophic, dilated, and restrictive cardiomyopathies because they have overlapping features and often mutate from one type to another during the course of the disease. Cardiomyopathies are then classified into 2 groups, *primary* when there is only heart involvement, and *secondary* if the heart is affected by systemic diseases with multiorganic involvement. (Table 1) *Primary cardiomyopathies* are divided into *genetic, acquired,* and *mixed* (genetic and acquired).

GENETIC	MIXED	ACQUIRED
Hypertrophic	Dilated	Inflammatory
Arrhythmogenic Right Ventricular	Restrictive	Tako-tsubo
Noncompaction		Peripartum
Glycogen Storage		Tachycardia-induced
Mitochondrial		Infants of diabetic mothers
Conduction Defects		
Ion Channelopathies		

Table 1. Classification of the primary cardiomyopathies (modified from B.J. Maron, et al., 2006a).

A salient feature of this classification is the inclusion of *ion channelopathies* caused by gene coding mutations of Na, K, and Ca channels. These channelopathies may result in deadly ventricular arrhythmias and can only be identified by molecular genetic studies since no structural cardiac damage is objectified. The Brugada syndrome, the long and short QT syndromes, the cathecolaminergic polymorphic ventricular tachycardia, and the unexplained nocturnal sudden death in Southeastern Asian youngsters belong to the channelopathies. Some conduction disorders are also included in the classification.

In contrast with the American Heart Association point of view, the European Society of Cardiology issued a report in the year 2008 with an updated definition and classification of the cardiomyopathies (Elliot et al., 2008). (Table 2) It was there stated that "Cardiomyopathies are structural and functional myocardial diseases in the absence of systemic hypertension, coronary atherosclerosis, valvulopathies, or congenital heart disease sufficient to explain the observed abnormality". Therefore, *hypertrophic cardiomyopathy* was defined as "Increased ventricular thickness or mass in the absence of loading conditions sufficient to cause the observed abnormality". This definition better reflects the terminology used in pediatrics (Elliot et al., 2008; Franklin et al., 1999). With regard to the classification, it was based on the identification of phenotypes according to their structural and functional features recognizing the following cardiomyopathies: *hypertrophic, dilated, restrictive, arrhythmogenic right ventricular, and unclassified* (Colan et al., 2007). Every phenotype could be *familial* or *non-familial* emphasizing the role of genetics in some cardiomyopathies and orienting the etiologic diagnosis. The differentiation between primary and secondary cardiomyopathy is then abandoned. *Left ventricular non-compaction* and the *takotsubo cardiomyopathy* are included in the group of unclassified cardiomyopathies. The European Society of Cardiology experts do not believe that *channelopathies* and *conduction disorders* should be considered as cardiomyopathies. In our opinion, the European Society of Cardiology classification is more user-friendly for general physicians.

CARDIOMYOPATHIES					
HCM	DCM		ARVC	RCM	Unclassified

FAMILIAL/	GENETIC	NON-FAMILIAL/	NON-GENETIC
Unidentified gene defect	Disease sub-type	Idiopathic	Disease sub-type

HCM: hypertrophic cardiomyopathy, DCM: dilated cardiomyopathy, ARVC: arrhythmogenic right ventricular cardiomyopathy, RCM: restrictive cardiomyopathy.

Table 2. European Society of Cardiology classification of primary cardiomyopathies (modified from Elliot, et al., 2008).

2. Classification

Though hypertrophic cardiomyopathy was first recognized by Liouville in France in 1869, (Liouville, 1869, as cited in Marian, 2007), it was not until the 1950's that was rediscovered in Britain by Brock and Teare (Brock & Fleming, 1956; Teare, 1958). Initial reports emphasized the presence of left ventricular outflow tract obstruction until it was realized that this could be absent (B. J. Maron et al, 2009). Since then, two main types of hypertrophic cardiomyopathy were distinguished, with or without obstruction. Nowadays, we know that hypertrophic cardiomyopathy, is the most frequent monogenic disorder in cardiology and the commonest cause of sudden death in youngsters in either form of presentation (J. Seidman & C. Seidman, 2001).

Regardless of the presence or absence of obstruction, hypertrophic cardiomyopathy is classified into two main groups, *familial* and *non-familial*. (Table 3) The latter comprises 4 subgroups: hypertrophic cardiomyopathy associated with *obesity, infants born to diabetic mothers, athlete's heart*, and *amyloidosis*. This chapter will mainly address the *familial forms* of hypertrophic cardiomyopathy also composed of 4 subgroups: *sarcomeric*, and 3 others in association with *malformation syndromes, inborn errors of metabolism*, and *neuromuscular disorders* (Elliot et al., 2008). The sarcomeric forms are the most frequent and have an autosomal dominant inheritance. They are caused by missence mutations of genes encoding the contractile proteins of the sarcomere. A mutation involves the change of a DNA base for another resulting in the replacement of an aminoacid in a polypeptide for another. Though readable, the meaning (sense) of the genetic message is changed. Considerable genetic and phenotypic heterogeneity is found in hypertrophic cardiomyopathy. In other words, different gene mutations may cause similar phenotypes or on the contrary, the same gene may result in dissimilar ones. The presence of modifying genes, like that encoding angiotensin II, environmental influences, gender, and associated conditions might explain some of these dissimilarities (Alcalai et al., 2008). About 20 genes carrying a great number of mutations have already been identified in hypertrophic cardiomyopathy (Kim et al., 2011). (Table 4) However, just 3 of them, beta-myosin heavy chain (*MYH7*), myosin binding protein C (*MYBPC3*), and troponin T (*TNNT2*) are responsible for almost 75% of the cases, thence, the remaining are rare. The genes involved in pediatric hypertrophic cardiomyopathy have a similar frequency and distribution as in adult patients (Kaski et al., 2009).

FAMILIAL	NON-FAMILIAL.
Sarcomeric	Associated with obesity
Associated with malformation syndromes	Infants born to diabetic mothers
Associated with inborn errors of metabolism	Athlete's heart
Associated with neuromuscular disorders	Amyloidosis

Table 3. Classification of the hypertrophic cardiomyopathies (modified from Elliot et al., 2008).

It has been suggested that the genotype might have an influence in the prognosis in hypertrophic cardiomyopathy. Patients with *MYH7* mutation would have more severe ventricular hypertrophy and present earlier in life, those with *TNNT2* would have less left ventricular hypertrophy but higher risk of sudden death, and late onset of the disease and favorable prognosis would be found in patients with *MYBPC3* mutation (Moolman et al., 1997; Niimura et al., 1998; Watkins et al., 1992). Nevertheless, a more recent study showed that regardless of the gene mutation, patients with a positive molecular genetic study, had a higher risk of cardiovascular death, stroke, worse functional class, diastolic and systolic left ventricular dysfunction, and that the long term outcome was worse for patients carrying more than one mutation. (Bos et al., 2009) The latter finding was not corroborated in children. (Kaski et al., 2009).

GENE	PROTEINS	GENE	PROTEINS
MYH7	β-Myosin heavy chain	TTN	Titin
MYH6	α-Myosin heavy chain	LBD3	LIM binding domain 3
MYBPC3	Cardiac myosin binding protein C	CSRP3	Muscle LIM protein
TNNT2	Cardiac troponin T	TCAP	Telethonin
TNNI3	Cardiac troponin I	VCL	Vinculin/metavinculin
TNNC1	Cardiac troponin C	ACTN2	α-Actinin 2
TPM1	α-Tropomyosin	MYOZ2	Myozenin 2
MYL3	Myosin essential light chain	JPH2	Junctophillin-2
MYL2	Myosin regulatory light chain	PLN	Phospholamban
ACTC	α-Cardiac actin		

Table 4. Susceptibility genes in hypertrophic cardiomyopathy (modified from Bos et al., 2009 & Kim et al., 2011).

3. Prevalence

The estimated prevalence of hypertrophic cardiomyopathy in the adult population as assessed by echocardiographic screening is 1:500 (B.J. Maron et al., 1995a). However, in pediatrics, the observed prevalence is much lower because hypertrophic cardiomyopathy usually has late gene expression. Large population registries from Australia and the US show a prevalence varying between 0.47 and 1.24:100,000 inhabitants and an occurrence of nearly 25% among all types of cardiomyopathies (Lipschultz et al., 2003; Nugent et al., 2003). In our institution, the incidence of hypertrophic cardiomyopathy was 1.1% for all children with heart disease attending the Division of Cardiology of the Children's Hospital (Bruno et al., 2002).

4. Pathology

4.1 Macroscopic findings

The gross anatomy generally shows severe left ventricular hypertrophy and small cavity size. (Fig. 1) The hypertrophy mainly involves the ventricular septum, and for this reason, one of the early denominations of the disease was *asymmetric septal hypertrophy* (Henry et al., 1973). Notwithstanding, hypertrophy may occur symmetrically or affect other segments like the posterior wall, and the apical or middle sections of the left ventricle (Falicov & Resnekov, 1977; Louie & Maron, 1987; Minami et al., 2011; Yamaguchi et al., 1979). Midventricular obstructive hypertrophic cardiomyopathy is more frequent in Asians with a prevalence of around 10% in tertiary centers and carries a higher risk for adverse events (B.J. Maron et al., 2003a; Minami et al., 2011). Patients with apical involvement are less commonly genotype positive than those with the more frequent variants of the disease but the affected genes are usually the same frequently found in the other patients (*MYBPC3 and MYH7*) (Gruner et al., 2011). In infants and children, the right ventricle can also be involved (Biagini et al., 2005).Almost 5% of patients with hypertrophic cardiomyopathy evolve to end stage dilated cardiomyopathy with

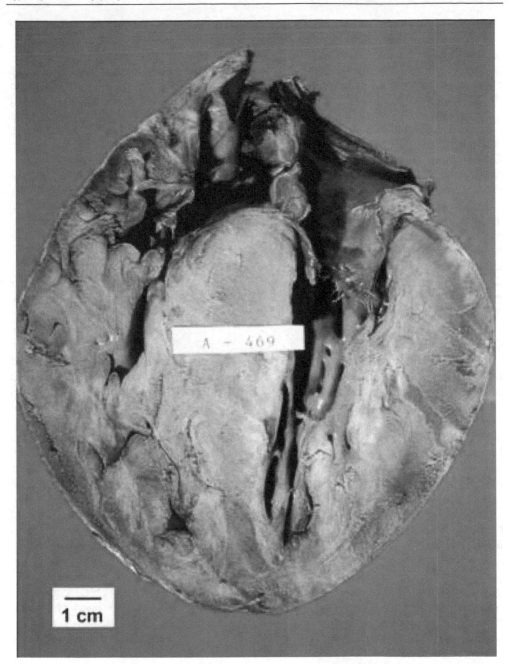

Fig. 1. Longitudinal section of the heart of a 9 year-old boy, who died suddenly during ordinary activities, with predominant hypertrophy of the septum but also showing increased thickness of the free wall of both ventricles. During life, obstruction of both the left and right ventricular outflow tracts was present.

extensive fibrosis, myocardial wall thinning and cavity dilation (Harris et al., 2006). The left atrium is enlarged as a consequence of the elevated left ventricular end diastolic pressure caused by diastolic dysfunction and mitral regurgitation secondary to left ventricular outflow tract obstruction or associated mitral valve anomalies (Klues et al., 1992). The physiopathology of mitral insufficiency in hypertrophic obstructive cardiomyopathy was initially attributed to the Venturi effect produced by systolic flow acceleration in the left ventricular outflow tract dragging the anterior mitral valve leaflet towards the ventricular septum causing both obstruction and insufficiency (Grigg et al., 1992; Panza et al., 1992; Shah et al., 1969 & 1971). A subsequent echocardiographic and Doppler study suggested instead, that the mitral valve leaflets are protruding into a narrow left ventricular outflow tract at the onset of ejection causing that rapid forward flow becomes the dominant force that pushes the leaflets toward the septum being the immediate cause of obstruction. After the onset of obstruction the leaflets are forced against the septum by the pressure difference across the orifice. The raising gradient leads to a smaller orifice and a higher gradient (Sherrid et al., 1993). The systolic anterior motion of the mitral leaflets precludes the proper sealing of the mitral orifice generating mild to moderate mitral regurgitation (M. Maron et al., 2011). The mitral valve in these patients shows alterations in size and shape which are thought to be primary abnormalities of the disease. The main changes are elongation and increase of the leaflet area usually not symmetrical. The size of the left ventricular outflow, the hyperdynamic contraction and the alterations of the mitral valve are the causes of the obstruction.

4.2 Microscopy

The distinct feature of the microscopic examination of the myocardium is hypertrophy and marked disarray (greater than 5% of the myocardial tissue) of individual and grouped myocardiocytes (myofibers) that instead of being normally aligned are interspersed in different directions forming whorls around areas of fibrosis. Cells and fibers lose their normal parallelism and can even be found almost perpendicular to each other. (Fig. 2) The disarray also includes the intracellular myofibrils. Other findings include increased connective tissue leading to interstitial fibrosis and thickening of the microvascular coronary artery walls with luminal reduction resulting in ischemia and fibrosis (Ferrans et al., 1972). Fibrosis and scar replacement of necrosed cells is more evident in areas with greater hypertrophy. Initially, it was postulated that the mechanism for the disarray and hypertrophy was caused by the increased effort of the myocytes to compensate the inefficient contractility of the affected sarcomere proteins. This would activate the insulin and tissue growth factors and angiotensin II resulting in the myocardial changes (J. Seidman & C. Seidman, 2001). Further experimental animal investigations and studies of hypertrophic cardiomyopathy mutations in man, by the same authors, found instead that the mutated sarcomeres had in fact increased function. It was then hypothesized that they would activate signals for hypertrophic remodeling. Abnormalities in calcium signaling were encountered leading to necrosis and replacement fibrosis producing diastolic dysfunction, a main feature of hypertrophic cardiomyopathy (C. Seidman & J. Seidman, 2011). An investigation by the same group, also found that a profibrotic marker like serum procollagen is significantly higher in patients with full blown hypertrophic cardiomyopathy and mutation carriers, with a still not developed phenotype, than in controls, pointing to increase collagen synthesis and fibrosis. Late gadolinium enhancement studies are positive when hypertrophy is already present (Ho et al., 2010). The myocardial disarray, interstitial fibrosis, and ischemia are also the substrate for the occurrence of arrhythmias.

4.3 Phenocopies

Patients with nonsarcomeric hypertrophic cardiomyopathy are considered to be phenocopies (Table 5), and might have the same pathologic findings as has been reported in some *malformation syndromes* or *neuromuscular disorders* like *Noonan's syndrome* and *Friedreich's ataxia* (Burch et al., 1992; Kawai et al., 2000). However, this is not the case for inborn *errors of metabolism* like *glycogen storage disease* where the gross anatomy resembles hypertrophic cardiomyopathy but microscopic examination shows the glycogen deposits in the myocytes without disarray. (Fig. 3) It should be noted that the present definition of phenocopy, according to the Webster's New World Medical Dictionary in its second acception is: "A person who has an environmental condition that mimics a condition that is produced by a gene". Since the examples just mentioned are genetic in origin, the term phenocopy could be inappropriate but is how these entities have been named for a long time.

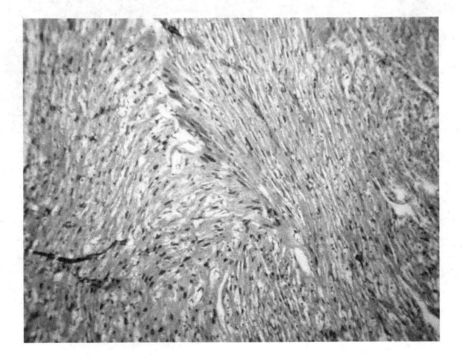

Fig. 2. Microscopic view of the myocardium with the typical disarray of hypertrophic cardiomyopathy in an infant who died in congestive heart failure. Myofibers have lost the usual parallel disposition and describe whorls around areas of fibrosis. The disarray is present in the myofibers, among myocytes and in the myofibrils within the myocytes.

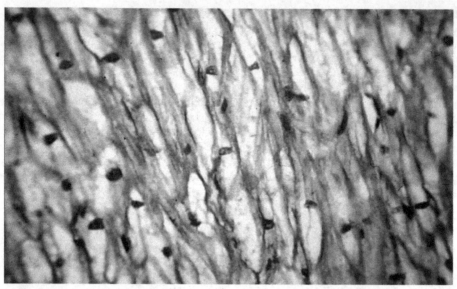

Fig. 3. Typical lacework appearance of the myocardium in a patient with type II Pompe's disease. There is normal alignment of the vacuolated myocardial fibers with glycogen storage.

GENE	PROTEIN	SYNDROME
TAZ	Tafazzin (G4.5)	Barth syndrome/LVNC
DTNA	α-dystrobrevin	Barth syndrome/LVNC
LAMP2	Lysosome-associated membrane protein 2	Danon's syndrome/WPW
GLA	α-galactosidase	Fabry's disease
AGL	Amylo-1,6-glucosidase	Forbes disease
FXN	Frataxin	Friedreich's ataxia
PTPN11	Protein tyrosine phosphatase. nonreceptor type 11, SHP-2	Noonan's syndrome, LEOPARD syndrome
RAF1	V-RAF-1 murine leukemia viral oncogene homolog 1	Noonan's syndrome, LEOPARD syndrome
KRAS	v-Ki-ras2 Kirsten rat sarcoma viral oncogene homolog	Noonan's syndrome
SOS1	Son of sevenless homolog 1	Noonan's syndrome
GAA	α-1,4-glucosidase deficiency	Pompe's disease
PRKAG2	AMP-activated protein kinase	WPW/HCM

LVNC: left ventricular noncompaction, WPW: Wolff-Parkinson-White, HCM: hypertrophic cardiomyopathy.

Table 5. Genes involved in the production of phenocopies (modified from Bos et al., 2009).

5. Clinical findings

Aside from the genetic and phenotypic heterogeneity already mentioned in hypertrophic cardiomyopathy, the age, form of presentation, and outcome, are also quite diverse. The age of the patient at presentation is a determinant of prognosis (Colan et al., 2007). Newborn and infants are more likely to be referred for congestive heart failure while older children are usually asymptomatic at the time of diagnosis and the consultation is requested because of the presence of a heart murmur, cardiomegaly casually detected on a chest x-ray, or electrocardiographic abnormalities (Bruno et al., 2002). Initially, asymptomatic patients may go on without symptoms for a long period of time until they begin experiencing fatigue and dyspnea, and less frequently, palpitations, chest pain, and syncope or sudden death which might be the first symptom ever. Another cause of referral is the investigation of cardiac involvement in patients with conditions known to be associated with hypertrophic cardiomyopathy like the *malformation syndromes, inborn errors of metabolism* or *neuromuscular disorders*. However, in other circumstances, the associated disease may have been unnoticed and the cardiomyopathy is discovered first. The presence of physical findings suggesting an association then prompts referral to the geneticist (Alday & Moreyra, 1984). With regard to the physical examination itself, in hypertrophic obstructive cardiomyopathy, the peripheral pulses may rise and descend rapidly. When considerable cardiac enlargement is present, a precordial bulge and outward displacement of the point of maximal impulse are usually found. A double apical impulse caused by a 4th heart sound is often noted. A harsh, blowing systolic murmur with varying intensity, related to the degree of obstruction and mitral regurgitation, can be listened along the left sternal border and at the apex. A distinctive feature of these murmurs is the variability seen with maneuvers that increase or reduce the obstruction intensifying or decreasing their intensity (Moreyra et al, 1972). (Fig. 4) Patients with non obstructive hypertrophic cardiomyopathy may also have ejection systolic murmurs along the left sternal border though softer than when there is left ventricular outflow obstruction. An ambulatory electrocardiographic study performed in infants, children and adolescents with hypertrophic cardiomyopathy concluded that arrhythmias occur rarely before adolescence. However, from then on, prevalence of nonsustained ventricular tachycardia is as high as 18%. It is also worth mentioning that absence of arrhythmias is not synonymous of low risk for sudden death (McKenna et al., 1988). Supraventricular and ventricular tachycardias may be equally found. Atrial fibrillation may occur in end-stage dilated hypertrophic cardiomyopathy (Harris et al., 2006). Very rarely, patients with hypertrophic cardiomyopathy have associated Wolff-Parkinson-White syndrome (Bockowski et al., 2007). The development of high rate supraventricular tachycardias is poorly tolerated in these patients with left ventricular diastolic dysfunction. This might lead to syncope and sudden death which are the most feared complications of hypertrophic cardiomyopathy. Several mechanisms have been reported as a cause of syncope like tachyarrhythmias, left ventricular outflow tract obstruction, systemic hypotension, and 3rd degree AV block. Sudden unexpected death may be the first and only symptom in hypertrophic cardiomyopathy and this is the most frequent cause of death in young athletes during competition. However, sudden death also occurs during usual activities, at rest, or during sleep time. The estimated rate of sudden death in children is 3% per year, a similar figure to that found in adults cared for in tertiary centers (Bruno & al., 2002; B.J. Maron et al., 1982; McKenna & Deanfield, 1984). Heart failure in this disease is usually provoked by diastolic dysfunction secondary to left ventricular hypertrophy, myocyte disarray and fibrosis. The presence of outflow obstruction is an additional factor leading to heart failure. In 3 to 5 % of patients the end stage is reached and systolic failure associated with left ventricular wall thinning and increased ventricular volume become a serious indication of poor prognosis (Biagini et al., 2005 & Harris et al., 2006).

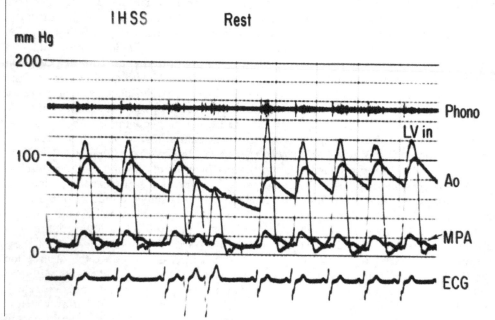

Fig. 4. Simultaneous hemodynamic recordings of the left ventricular inflow (LV in), aorta (Ao) and main pulmonary artery (MPA). An electrocardiogram (ECG) and a phonocardiogram (phono) were also recorded. There is a small basal gradient between the left ventricular inflow and the aorta which increases in a post-extrasystolic beat together with the intensity of the systolic murmur shown in the phonocardiogram, as a consequence of the stronger contraction following the post-extrasystolic pause. (IHSS: idiopathic hypertrophic subaortic stenosis).

6. Laboratory studies

6.1 Radiology

The chest x-ray is usually normal in early stages of the disease but following the pubertal growth spurt shows cardiomegaly at the expense of the left sided chambers (B.J. Maron et al., 1986). (Fig. 5) The same is true for patients evolving to end-stage hypertrophic cardiomyopathy (Biagini et al., 2005). Finally, infants with severe heart failure nearly always have considerable cardiac enlargement at presentation. Pulmonary venous hypertension secondary to elevation of the left ventricular end diastolic pressure is reflected by the well known resultant pulmonary vascular changes.

6.2 Electrocardiography and allied techniques

The electrocardiogram is usually abnormal in almost all patients with hypertrophic cardiomyopathy. (Panza & Maron, 1989) The electrocardiographic abnormality, even a slight one, may precede the echocardiographic findings showing left ventricular hypertrophy in family members carrying the genotype of probands with hypertrophic cardiomyopathy. Therefore, this should be kept on mind when screening relatives of hypertrophic cardiomyopathy patients (Gregor et al., 1989). Left atrial enlargement and left ventricular hypertrophy by voltage criteria usually associated with ST-T abnormalities are seen. (Fig. 6) Younger patients may have combined ventricular or isolated right ventricular hypertrophy with a rightwards QRS axis. (Fig. 7) Another frequent finding is the presence of pathological deep and narrow Q waves. An R + S sum higher than 10 mV on the limb leads of the electrocardiogram has been recently proposed as a risk factor for sudden death in children with hypertrophic cardiomyopathy (Ostman-Smith et al., 2005). (Fig. 8) An electrocardiographic Wolff-Parkinson-White pattern or syndrome is very rare in patients with sarcomeric hypertrophic cardiomyopathy. However, it has been described in mutations of genes like those encoding AMP-activated protein kinase (*PRKAG2*) and lysosome associated membrane protein 2 (*LAMP2*) producing *glycogen storage disease* and *Danon disease* respectively. Both of them recognized as phenocopies of hypertrophic cardiomyopathy (Alday et al., 2010). Ambulatory electrocardiography and exercise testing are used for arrhythmia detection and risk stratification in older children with hypertrophic cardiomyopathy. The presence of nonsustained ventricular tachycardia by Holter monitoring or an abnormal blood pressure response to exercise are considered risk factors for sudden death (Elliot et al., 2000).

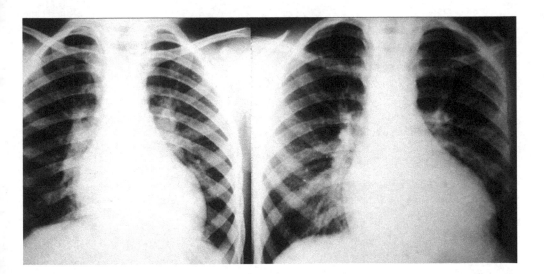

Fig. 5. Chest x-rays of a boy at 11 and 13 years of age showing great increase in the heart size coincident with pubertal growth spurt.

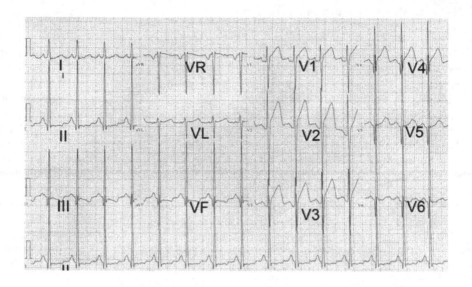

Fig. 6. Electrocardiogram of a 16 year-old male patient showing increased R wave voltages and secondary ST-T changes indicating severe left ventricular hypertrophy.

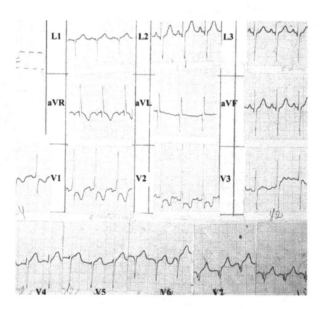

Fig. 7. Electrocardiogram belonging to a 4 year-old boy with a QRS axis of -120° with Q waves in leads II, III and aVF. There are signs of combined ventricular hypertrophy, loss of R wave voltage from V4 to V8 with appearance of QS complexes in V6 and pathological Q waves in V7 and V8.

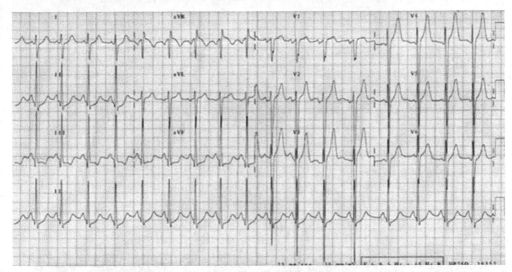

Fig. 8. Electrocardiogram of a 14 year-old male patient with a vertical QRS axis (+120°) and voltage criteria for left ventricular hypertrophy. A limb lead voltage sum > 10 mV is considered a risk factor for sudden death in children.

6.3 Echocardiography

Echocardiography associated with color flow Doppler is the most effective test for the diagnosis of hypertrophic cardiomyopathy (B.J. Maron et al., 2003a). It allows detection of the disease, follow-up of progression, and risk stratification for sudden death (B.J. Maron et al., 1986, Ostman-Smith et al., 2005). The wall thickness echocardiographic criteria for the diagnosis of hypertrophic cardiomyopathy was set at greater than 2 SD above the mean for the body surface area of the population for a localized or general myocardial hypertrophy (Grenier et al., 2000). When in the absence of pulmonary valve stenosis the right ventricular wall thickness exceeds 4 mm the right ventricle is considered to be involved too (Nugent et al., 2005). Left ventricular hypertrophy is most frequently asymmetric with greater involvement of the interventricular septum than the rest of the walls, though it can also be concentric. (Fig. 9 - 11) More rarely, it is localized in the anterior wall, the apex, or in the mid left ventricle (M. Maron et al., 2009, Minami et al., 2011). The mid ventricular obstruction may lead to the development of an apical left ventricular aneurysm. (Fig. 12) In younger children the right ventricle may also be affected (Biagini et al., 2005). As a consequence of mitral insufficiency and/or diastolic dysfunction, there is left atrial enlargement. The systolic anterior movement of the mitral valve contacting the ventricular septum that causes left ventricular outflow tract obstruction in patients with hypertrophic obstructive cardiomyopathy is readily seen (B.J. Maron et al., 2003). Color flow mapping allows detection of the site of obstruction. (Fig. 13) The gradient across the outflow tract is estimated by continuous wave Doppler that also allows assessment of the mitral regurgitation severity. (Fig. 14) Transesophageal echocardiography is more sensitive than transthoracic studies for evaluation of primary mitral valve anomalies producing mitral incompetence (Kuhl & Hanrath, 2004). The presence of left ventricular outflow tract obstruction is now considered a risk factor for adverse events in hypertrophic cardiomyopathy (M. Maron et al., 2003). Furthermore, we now know that almost 70% of patients with hypertrophic cardiomyopathy have gradients across the left ventricular outflow considering the obstruction caused by exercise, when studied with stress echo. Actually, it should be performed in all patients with no significant gradient at rest (M. Maron et al., 2006). Estimation of diastolic dysfunction in hypertrophic cardiomyopathy is performed by studying the pulmonary vein and transmitral Doppler flow tracings but since they depend on loading conditions are not reliable to predict adverse outcomes in children with hypertrophic cardiomyopathy (McMahon et al., 2004). Tissue Doppler velocities measurements at the mitral annulus level are more sensitive in detecting diastolic dysfunction allowing early diagnosis in hypertrophic cardiomyopathy genetic carriers before they develop hypertrophy (Nagheb et al., 2003). (Fig. 15) Tissue Doppler studies can also predict adverse events like death, ventricular tachycardia, cardiac arrest, and exercise intolerance in affected children with the disease (McMahon et al., 2004).

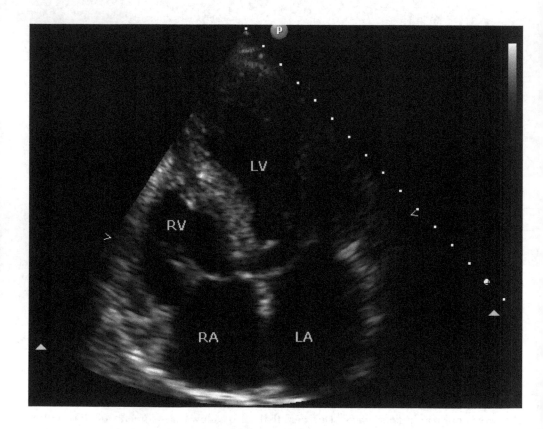

Fig. 9. Four-chamber bidimensional echocardiographic view of a 16 year-old asymptomatic male patient with hypertrophic cardiomyopathy with asymmetric septal hypertrophy. The septum and the posterior wall measure 21 mm and 9.5 mm respectively.

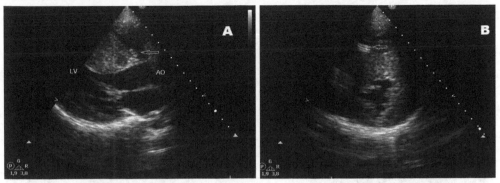

Fig. 10. Bidimensional echocardiogram showing long (A) and short (B) axis parasternal views of the left ventricle of a 22 year-old female followed since early childhood with severe asymmetrical hypertrophy of the septum measuring 31 mm in diameter. There is convexity toward the left ventricular cavity. The mitral leaflets initiate an anterior motion to provoke mitral septal contact and the resultant left ventricular outflow tract obstruction. The left atrium is mildly enlarged. The tip of a catheter for DDD pacing is seen in the right ventricular cavity (arrows).

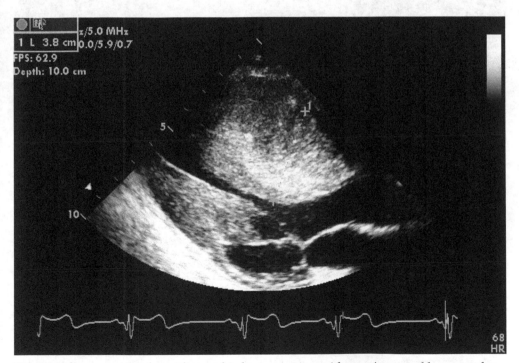

Fig. 11. Bidimensional echocardiographic long axis view with massive septal hypertrophy (38 mm) in a girl with a strong family history (2 siblings). Courtesy Dr Ricardo Pignatelli, Texas Children's Hospital.

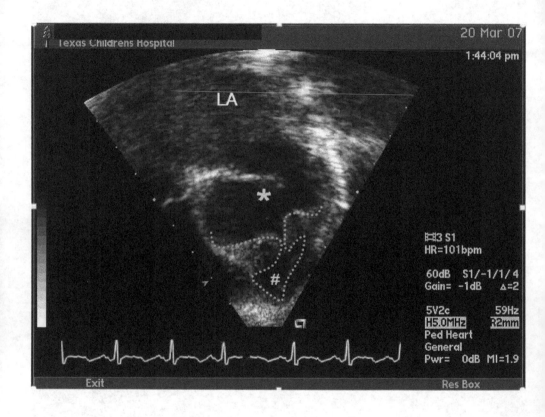

Fig. 12. Bidimensional echocardiographic view of a patient with midventricular obstruction. The left ventricle has an upper inflow (*) and a lower apical chamber (#) as a result of the obstruction. Courtesy Dr Ricardo Pignatelli, Texas Children's Hospital.

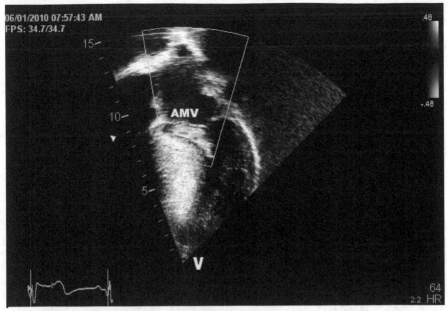

Fig. 13. Echocardiographic 4-chamber view of asymmetric septal hypertrophy with left ventricular outflow tract flow acceleration (arrow) by color Doppler. (AMV: anterior mitral valve). Courtesy Dr Ricardo Pignatelli, Texas Children's Hospital.

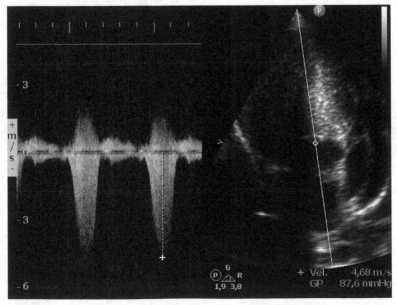

Fig. 14. Continuous wave Doppler showing a severe gradient (87.6 mmHg) across the left ventricular outflow tract in the same patient shown on figure 10.

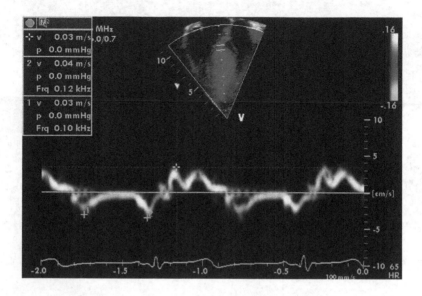

Fig. 15. Decreased Doppler tissue septal velocities (<5cm/second) in a patient with massive hypertrophic cardiomyopathy. Courtesy Dr Ricardo Pignatelli, Texas Children's Hospital.

6.4 Computed tomography and magnetic resonance imaging

Cardiac computed tomography and magnetic resonance imaging yield superior anatomic data than echocardiography since they allow better definition of the anterolateral wall and tip of the left ventricle and the right ventricle. However, these procedures are more costly and the former exposes the patient to radiation (M. Maron et al., 2009). (Fig. 16) Nevertheless, they are very useful when thoracic deformities prevent satisfactory cardiac visualization by transthoracic echocardiography. Cardiovascular magnetic resonance has also demonstrated that mitral leaflet elongation is present in hypertrophic cardiomyopathy independently of other phenotypic variants indicating that the mitral abnormalities are primary, thus, their important role in the pathophysiology of the left ventricular outflow obstruction (M. Maron, et al.; 2011). On the other hand, gadolinium magnetic resonance imaging late enhancement allows detection of the amount of myocardial fibrosis and is a predictor of systolic dysfunction (M. Maron et al., 2008). A more recent study reports that is also effective for prognostication of adverse outcomes and which patients might require a cardioverter-defibrillator (Fig. 17) (Bruder et al., 2010).

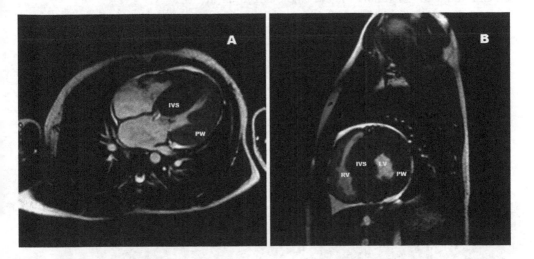

Fig. 16. A. Long axis view of a cardiac magnetic resonance image of a 5 year-old asymptomatic boy with severe hypertrophic cardiomyopathy. **B:** Magnetic resonance imaging of a short axis projection of the heart of a 3 year-old boy with severe heart failure. (IVS: interventricular septum, LV: left ventricle, PW: posterior wall, RV: right ventricle). Courtesy Dr Ricardo Pignatelli, Texas Children's Hospital.

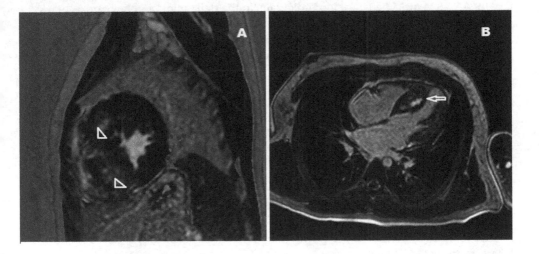

Fig. 17. **A.** Cardiac magnetic resonance image of the heart of a patient with positive delayed gadolinium enhancement indicating a diffuse pattern of fibrosis (arrowheads). **B:** Long axis view of a cardiac magnetic resonance image of the heart of a 9 year-old boy with a localized delayed gadolinium enhancement image in the interventricular septum (arrow). Courtesy Dr Ricardo Pignatelli, Texas Children's Hospital.

6.5 Cardiac catheterization and cineangiocardiography

We owe to cardiac catheterization and cineangiocardiography the initial understanding of the physiopathology of hypertrophic cardiomyopathy shortly after its rediscovery about half a century ago (Braunwald et al., 1964; Wigle, Auger & Marquis, 1967). These techniques were then considered the gold standard for the diagnosis of hypertrophic obstructive cardiomyopathy. (Fig. 18) With the advent of the just discussed noninvasive imaging techniques like Doppler-echocardiography, computed tomography, and magnetic resonance imaging, this invasive procedure is no longer necessary for diagnostic purposes. Nowadays, this method is only used before planned surgical treatment or percutaneous interventions for septal reduction.

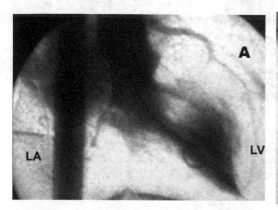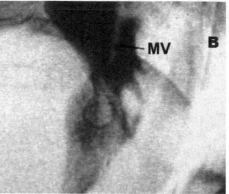

Fig. 18. A. Left ventricular cineangiocardiogram in the right anterior oblique projection showing a hypertrophied chamber with subaortic obstruction and moderate mitral insufficiency with left atrial enlargement. B. In the left anterior oblique view the anterior mitral valve can be seen contacting the septum. LV: left ventricle; LA: left atrium; MV: mitral valve.

7. Complications

7.1 Sudden death and congestive heart failure

The main complications in children with hypertrophic cardiomyopathy are syncope and sudden unexpected death. The latter may be the first and only manifestation of the disease and is considered to be secondary to ventricular tachycardia and fibrillation caused by myocardial fibrosis and ischemia (Basso et al., 2000; B.J. Maron et al., 2000b). Sudden death occurs more often in older children with hypertrophic cardiomyopathy either during strenuous sport activities or at rest but is infrequent in infants (B.J. Maron et al., 2003a) who are more prone to present and die with congestive heart failure specially in secondary forms (Bruno et al., 2002).

7.2 Arrhythmias

Supraventricular and nonsustained ventricular tachycardias, were found in almost a third of pediatric and adolescent patients with hypertrophic cardiomyopathy studied by ambulatory electrocardiography (McKenna, et al., 1988). However, their outcome after a mean follow-up of 3 years was rather benign. In a study from our group, a quarter of the patients had symptomatic atrial or ventricular tachycardia. Three out of 7 died suddenly during follow-up (Bruno et al., 2002). Rarely, 3rd degree atrioventricular block is found in children with hypertrophic cardiomyopathy. They could present with near syncope or syncopal attacks as the 1st manifestation of the disease (Rosen et al., 1997).

7.3 Evolving phenotype
Children with hypertrophic cardiomyopathy may evolve to dilated or restrictive cardiomyopathy phenotypes in 5% of the cases. In both circumstances they have a dimmer prognosis and become candidates for heart transplantation (Biagini et al., 2005; Denfield et al., 1997; Shirani et al., 1993).

7.4 Infectious endocarditis
Bacterial endocarditis is an uncommon complication in hypertrophic cardiomyopathy though can occur affecting the left ventricular aspect of the anterior mitral valve leaflet, especially in the presence of obstruction (Aoun et al., 1994; Morgan-Hughes & Motwani, 2002). Antibiotic prophylaxis for infectious endocarditis is then recommended.

7.5 Stroke
Ischemic stroke is somewhat frequent and a cause of death in adult hypertrophic cardiomyopathy but has not been mentioned in children (B.J. Maron et al., 2000a).

8. Differential diagnosis

The most important differential diagnosis is with the athlete's heart and is sometimes somewhat difficult to make. Highly trained competitive athletes may have electrocardiographic abnormalities that resemble those of hypertrophic cardiomyopathy. As in this situation, the left ventricle is hypertrophied but the wall thickness as determined by echocardiography does not exceed 15 mm in diameter and the hypertrophy is symmetrical. The left ventricular cavity is dilated and the ejection fraction is normal while hypertrophic cardiomyopathy is frequently accompanied by unusual distribution of hypertrophy, the left ventricle is smaller in size (<4.5 cm) and the ejection fraction is higher than normal. Furthermore, left ventricular diastolic function is normal in young athletes but is always impaired in hypertrophic cardiomyopathy (B.J. Maron, Spirito & Pelliccia, 1995b). Tissue Doppler studies has also been very useful to distinguish those patients in the "grey zone" (Cardim et al., 2003). When still in doubt regarding the diagnosis, cessation of physical activities usually results in regression of the left ventricular mass in a few weeks' time (B.J. Maron et al.., 1993). Genetic screening might be useful when they are positive for a mutation which occurs in up to 70% of patients with hypertrophic cardiomyopathy. On the contrary, a negative test does not exclude the possibility of a mutation still not discovered.

9. Phenocopies and associations

A recent large epidemiologic study of the pediatric population with hypertrophic cardiomyopathy established that almost a quarter of patients with unexplained left ventricular hypertrophy do not have a sarcomeric etiology (Colan et al., 2007). These variants are called phenocopies and are listed in Table 5. They are classified as *malformation syndromes, inborn errors of metabolism, and neuromuscular disorders* and each group numbers about one third of the total.

9.1 Malformation syndromes
9.1.1 Noonan's and LEOPARD syndromes
The most common *malformation syndromes* associated with hypertrophic cardiomyopathy included in the European Society of Cardiology classification of familial hypertrophic cardiomyopathy, are Noonan's syndrome and its allelic variant LEOPARD syndrome, acronym for lentiginosis, electrocardiographic anomalies, ocular hypertelorism, pulmonic stenosis, abnormal male genitalia, retardation of growth, and deafness. The prevalence of Noonan,s syndrome, initially described as the Turner phenotype with normal karyotype (Noonan, 1968), is estimated in 1:2,000 births (Nora et al., 1974). (Fig. 19) It is inherited as an autosomic dominant form and nearly 80% have congenital heart disease, most frequently pulmonic valve and arterial stenoses, and atrial and ventricular septal defects. The introduction of echocardiography as a diagnostic tool, allowed the recognition of an association with hypertrophic cardiomyopathy in almost a quarter of patients (Nora et al., (1975). In the Australian epidemiologic study of childhood cardiomyopathies, 28% of 80 patients with hypertrophic cardiomyopathy had Noonan's syndrome (Nugent et al., 2005). These patients presented earlier and had more frequent biventricular involvement. However, they did not find greater adverse events rate than in sarcomeric hypertrophic cardiomyopathy. In about 40-50% of patients a mutation of protein tyrosine phosphatase nonreceptor type 11 (*PTPN11*) is found (Type 1 Noonan's syndrome), but this is present in 90% of LEOPARD patients (Sznajer et al., 2007; Tartaglia et al., 2001). This gene controls a series of developmental processes, among them the genesis of semilunar valves. The mutation is then mainly present in patients with heart defects but not in those with hypertrophic cardiomyopathy.

9.1.2 Related conditions
Some related genetic conditions to Noonan's syndrome like the Costello syndrome, the cardiofaciocutaneous syndrome, and palmo-plantar hyperkeratosis with woolly hair may also be associated with hypertrophic cardiomyopathy (Peirone et al., 2005, Roberts et al., 2006).

9.2 Inborn errors of metabolism
9.2.1 Pompe's disease
Pompe's disease or type II glycogen storage disease is an autosomal recessive inherited disorder caused by absence of the acid alpha-glucosidase enzyme (*GAA*) preventing the normal degradation of glycogen in the cardiac myocyte (Hers, 1963). There is an infantile type with massive cardiac enlargement as seen in hypertrophic cardiomyopathy with obstruction leading to congestive heart failure and early death (Ehlers et al., 1962). A typical electrocardiogram is shown in Fig. 20. Late onset Pompe's disease with a better outcome has also been described (Winkle et al., 2005). Enzyme replacement therapy is now available for treatment of *GAA* deficiency.

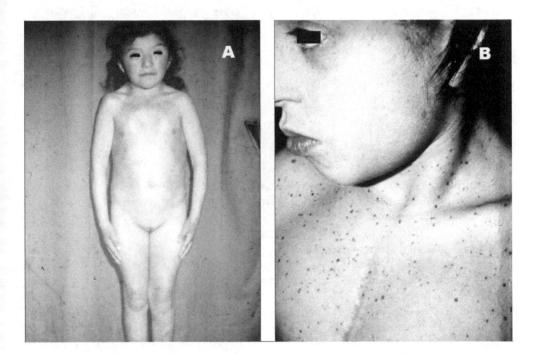

Fig. 19. **A.** Phenotype of a 10-year-old girl with Noonan's syndrome and hypertrophic cardiomyopathy. There is short stature, peculiar face, eyelid ptosis with downward slant, ocular and mammillar hypertelorism, low set ears, pterigium colli, and a prominent chest. **B.** Ten-year-old girl with LEOPARD syndrome. The multiple lentigines and hypertrophic obstructive cardiomyopathy became apparent long after she had been operated on for severe pulmonary valve stenosis when she was 6-month old (Reproduced with permission from *Am Heart J,* 1984; Vol.108, pp. 996-1000).

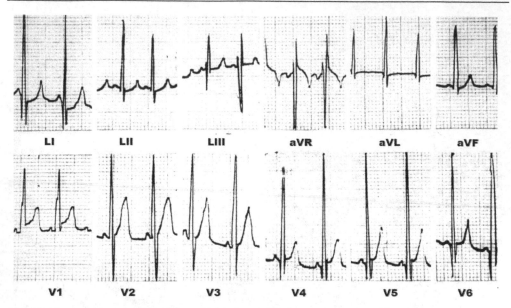

| LI | LII | LIII | aVR | aVL | aVF |

| V1 | V2 | V3 | V4 | V5 | V6 |

Fig. 20. Typical electrocardiogram of an infant with Pompe's disease. There is short atrioventricular conduction and biventricular hypertrophy with large voltages and no repolarization abnormalities.

9.2.2 Other glycogen storage diseases

A genetic study of 75 patients with hypertrophic cardiomyopathy found that 3 out of 35 patients with negative sarcomere protein mutations had genetical defects in lysosome-associated membrane protein 2 (*LAMP2*) responsible for the X-linked disorder   Danon's disease/Wolff-Parkinson-White in 2 of the 3, and in AMP-activated protein kinase gamma 2 (*PRKAG2*) in the remaining, causing Wolff-Parkinson-White/hypertrophic cardiomyopathy (Arad et al., 2005). Both conditions produce glycogen storage and might wrongly be considered as sarcomeric hypertrophic cardiomyopathies. The presence of preexcitation should point to the correct diagnosis. Type IIIa and IV glycogen storage diseases are very rare conditions caused by deficiencies in debrancher and branching enzymes respectively. These patients have muscular hypotonia with elevated creatine kinase and heart and liver involvement. There is heterogenous severity of the disease and the hypertrophic cardiomyopathy is concentric. The inheritance is autosomal recessive (Kishnani et al., 2010). (Fig. 21)

9.2.3 Fabry's disease

Fabry's disease, an X-linked disorder characterized by intracellular accumulation of glycosphingolipids caused by deficiency of the lysosomal enzyme alpha-galactoside A (*GLA*) may result in late onset hypertrophic cardiomyopathy, therefore it is rare in children. The reported prevalences in adult males and females with hypertrophic cardiomyopathy are 7.5 and 12% respectively (Chimenti et al., 2004; Sachdev et al., 2002). Enzyme replacement therapy for these patients is available (Eng et al., 2001).

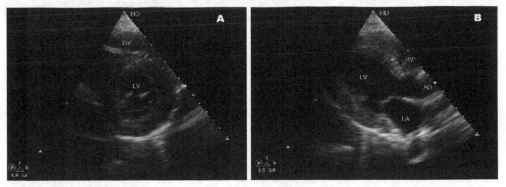

Fig. 21. Short and long axis parasternal echocardiographic views of the heart of a 19-year-old female with type III glycogen storage disease with concentric hypertrophic cardiomyopathy.

9.3 Neuromuscular disorders

Friedreich's ataxia is an autosomic recessive hereditary disorder with spinocerebellar degeneration and frequently associated with hypertrophic cardiomyopathy (Gottdiener et al., 1982). A mutation of the frataxin gene (*FXN*) alters the energy production through mitochondrial iron dysmetabolism resulting in mitochondrial damage producing muscle fiber fibrosis (Michael et al., 2006). The cardiomyopathy may precede the neurological manifestations (Alday & Moreyra, 1984).

9.4 Association with congenital heart disease

Not infrequently, hypertrophic cardiomyopathy and congenital heart disease are associated in children (Somerville & Becu, 1978). In most circumstances the defects are not severe. Ventricular and atrial septal defects and pulmonary valve stenosis have been reported, the last two mainly in patients with Noonan's and LEOPARD syndromes (Bruno et al., 2002; Tikanoja et al., 1999). However, associations with severe conditions like tetralogy of Fallot and atrioventricular septal defect have also been found (Alday et al., 1985; Eidem et al., 2000). (Fig. 22)

9.5 Association with left ventricular noncompaction

Left ventricular noncompaction belongs to the category of unclassified cardiomyopathies . It is characterized by presence of prominent myocardial trabeculations and sinusoid tracts mainly in the left ventricle. (Fig. 23) Affected patients frequently develop a dilated cardiomyopathy with heart failure, arrhythmias, and systemic thromboembolism. Recent molecular studies have shown that mutations of genes producing phenocopies like Barth syndrome, or even dilated and hypertrophic cardiomyopathies, are present in patients with left ventricular noncompaction. We recently reported a family with overlapping phenotypes for left ventricular noncompaction, hypertrophic cardiomyopathy, and Wolff- Parkinson-White syndrome. We could not obtain genetic molecular studies but on the basis of features shared with affected patients suspected a mutation of either *PRKG2 and LAMP-2* which cause hypertrophic cardiomyopathy with Wolff-Parkinson-White syndrome or Danon's disease respectively (Alday et al., 2010).

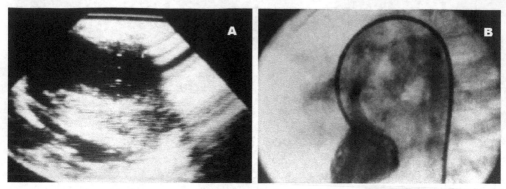

Fig. 22. Two dimensional echocardiogram (A) and left ventricular cineangiography (B) in a patient with tetralogy of Fallot six months after a right modified Blalock-Taussig shunt showing severe ventricular septal hypertrophy, a hypoplastic left ventricle and a dilated aorta overriding a ventricular septal defect.

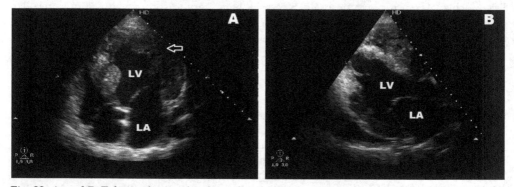

Fig. 23. A and B. Echocardiographic four-chamber view of two sisters followed since infancy showing hypertrophic cardiomyopathy and associated left ventricular noncompaction. The arrow in A points deep sinusoid tracts. LV: left ventricle, LA: left atrium.

10. Treatment

The treatment of hypertrophic cardiomyopathy aims to improve the quality of life alleviating symptoms and to stratify the risk for sudden death to prevent it from happening. Several algorrhythms have been proposed, a slightly modified one is shown in Fig. 24 (Berger et al., 2009). These authors emphasize the existing difficulties to implement prospective controlled randomized trials to define the benefits of different treatment options for this population, therefore most current therapies are empirical or the result of consensus. In older children intensive physical exercise is contraindicated. The disease presenting early has a severe prognosis this being the reason for indicating medical treatment even in asymptomatic children (Bruno et al., 2002). Patients who are symptomatic should receive pharmacological treatment with adrenergic beta blockers which do not decrease the basal outflow gradient but are able to prevent its accentuation in situations of exacerbated inotropism of the heart.

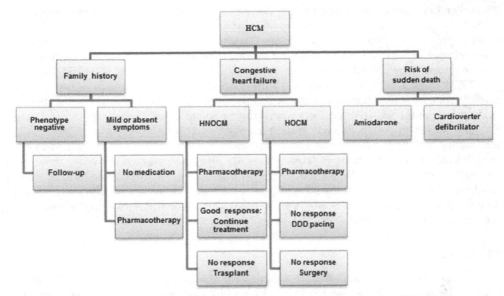

Fig. 24. Algorithm for the treatment of hypertrophic cardiomyopathy (Modified from Berger, et al. (2009) *Cardiol Young,* Vol.19, pp. 66-73).

Beta blockers also have anti-ischemic properties which increase ventricular filling by decreasing the heart rate. In these patients, calcium channel blockers like verapamil can be an alternative to beta blockers. It is not recommended to use them together. In patients with severe gradients and pulmonary hypertension are not advised because of the danger of precipitating acute pulmonary edema. If there is no improvement, disopyramide, which is an antiarrhythmic drug with negative inotropic effects, is able to decrease basal gradients. The combination of disopyramide and beta blockers has been used succesfully in adults but there is no reported experience in children (Sherrid et al., (2005). For very symptomatic smaller children, in spite of full medical treatment, permanent DDD pacing with short atrioventricular interval to favor the consistent capture of the right ventricle has been used to lower the left ventricular outflow tract obstruction by changing the pattern of left ventricular activation (Alday et al., 1998 & Fananapazir et al., 1992). DDD pacing is a reasonable alternative to surgery in symptomatic children despite pharmacological treatment if they are still too young for surgery, taking into account that the approach to an extended septal myectomy is just the aortic valve with a small annulus at this age. A very recent study has also shown progressive relief of symptoms and gradient reduction at long term follow-up (Galve et al., 2010). However, as with other types of treatment, DDD pacing does not protect against the possibility of sudden arrhythmic death (Bruno et al., 2002). The gold standard for the treatment of hypertrophic obstructive cardiomyopathy is still the surgical septal myomectomy (B.J. Maron et al., 2003a; Stone et al., 1993). In experienced centers the mortality is very low and the abolition of the gradient is instantaneous and persistent. The remaining obstruction is usually negligible. These excellent hemodynamic results are associated with improvement of symptoms. The results have been followed for many years and the need for repeat procedures is rare. It should be remembered that the child has to be old enough to permit the transaortic approach to the septum (Berger et al.,

2009). For this reason, reoperation might be necessary in children 14-year-old or younger (Minakata et al., 2005). With regard to catheter septal ablation with alcohol or radiofrequency the 2003 Expert Consensus Document on Hypertrophic Cardiomyopathy, addressing alcohol septal ablation, states that until the long-term effects of the myocardial scar are known, the procedure is not advised in children (Jensen et al., 2011; B.J. Maron et al., 2003a; Sigwart 1995) In patients with symptomatic hypertrophic nonobstructive cardiomyopathy, calcium antagonists like verapamil could be used to improve the diastolic performance of the left ventricle. Beta blockers are also indicated in this form of the disease. Recently the use of perhexiline which is a metabolic modulator has been introduced for the treatment of patients with this phenotype with improvement of the diastolic performance of the left ventricle and of symptoms (Abozguia et al.; 2010). This was a preliminary report that has still to be supported by further investigations. Infants with heart failure and older children with evolution to a dilated cardiomyopathy should be treated with drugs usually employed for treatment of systolic heart failure. These cases may eventually need heart transplantation (Shirani et al., 1993).

11. Prevention

Risk stratification of sudden death in infants and children differs from what is done in adults. In children, cardiac death occurs infrequently and non sudden cardiac death is as common as sudden arrhythmic death. The main risk factors for sudden death in children with hypertrophic cardiomyopathy are, according to Maron et al., previous cardiac arrest, syncope, or sustained ventricular tachycardia, family history of sudden death, frequent repetitive non sustained ventricular tachycardia, abnormal blood pressure response to exercise, end-stage hypertrophic cardiomyopathy, and massive left ventricular hypertrophy (B.J. Maron et al., 2003b). Other criteria for death prognostication proposed more recently, specifically in children, take into account the electrocardiographic voltage and echocardiographic parameters like the septal thickness and the left ventricular wall/left ventricular diastolic dimension ratio (Ostman-Smith et al., 2005). For non-sudden cardiac death, massive left ventricular hypertrophy and abnormal blood pressure response to exercise are considered significant risk factors for mortality (Decker et al., 2009). Sudden cardiac death due to hypertrophic cardiomyopathy occurs mostly in adolescence and early adulthood and very infrequently before 10 years of age. These cases are due to ventricular tachycardia or ventricular fibrillation. In fact, hypertrophic cardiomyopathy is the most common cause of sudden death in the young including athletes (J. Seidman & C. Seidman, 2001). This is the reason why the diagnosis of hypertrophic cardiomyopathy at this age is a strong indication to discontinue the practice of competitive sports. At this time it seems that to establish a prognosis by the knowledge of the specific disease causing mutation is not reasonable for the individual patient. Implantable cardioverter defibrillators are effective to prevent arrhythmic sudden death but in infants and children are indicated mainly in secondary prevention (B.J. Maron, et al., 2000b; Epstein, A.; et al., 2008). The cardioverter defibrillator implantation is plagued with complications in children, this being the reason for the reluctance of its use in primary prevention (Berul et al., 2008). In a nonrandomized controlled trial amiodarone was at one time reported to improve survival in hypertrophic cardiomyopathy associated with ventricular tachycardia (McKenna et al., 1985). However, the frequent toxic effects of amiodarone might counteract its benefits (Berger et al., 2009). It then could be concluded that the properly functioning cardioverter defibrillator is nowadays the only effective treatment for the prevention of sudden arrhythmic death (B.J. Maron, et al., 2000b).

12. Screening strategies

It is well known that hypertrophic cardiomyopathy is a genetic disease of the sarcomeric proteins with great heterogeneity of genetic basis and fenotypic expression which does not only involve these structures but also include abnormalities of the connective tissue, mitral valve, and intramural coronary arteries. The genetic defect may be influenced by modifiers genes and unknown enviromental factors. The strategy for clinical screening for hypertrophic cardiomyopathy with 12 lead electrocardiogram and echocardiogram in non affected family members including < 12 year-old children, is optional, unless there is history of early death due to hypertrophic cardiomyopathy or other serious complications in the family, or is an athlete in training, or evidence of incipient left ventricular hypertrophy, or onset of suspicious symptoms. In family members 12 to 18 years of age, clinical follow-up should be performed every 12 to 18 months and from then on every 5 years. The period of screening should be extended to adulthood since we now know that certain mutant genes can provoke a disease of rather late onset (B.J. Maron et al., 2004).

13. Conclusion

Great strides have been made since the rediscovery of hypertrophic cardiomyopathy in the late 50's last century. Important advances in the understanding of the genetics and physiopathology of the disease have occurred as well as development of superb imaging technologies. Treatment is tailored according to the phenotype and stage of the disease. The very important differences between adult and childhood hypertrophic cardiomyopathy have been underlined in this chapter hoping that will help physicians in decision making when dealing with these patients.

14. Aknowledgement

We thank Professor Ricardo Pignatelli from Texas Children's Hospital for providing us with excellent images from his personal archives and helpful advice.
We also thank Mr. Alfredo Benito from Photographic Resources for helping us with the artwork, and Dr. Ana Grassani for her assistance in the preparation of the manuscript.
Finally, we thank our patients for trusting us for many years.

15. References

[1] Abozguia, K.; Elliott, P.; McKenna, W.; et al. (2010). Metabolic modulator perhexiline corrects energy deficiency and improves exercise capacity in symptomatic hypertrophic cardiomyopathy. *Circulation*, Vol.122, pp. 1562-9.

[2] Alcalai, R.; Seidmann, J. & Seidman, C. (2008). Genetic basis of hypertrophic cardiomyopathy from bench to the clinic. *Cardiovasc Electrophysiol*, Vol.19, pp. 104-110.

[3] Alday, L.; Moreyra, E. (1984). Secondary hypertrophic cardiomyopathy in infancy and childhood. *Am Heart J*, Vol.108, pp. 996-1000.

[4] Alday, L.; Moreyra, E.; Juaneda, E.; et al. (1985). Hypertrophic cardiomyopathy in a child with tetralogy of Fallot. *J Cardiovasc Ultrasonography*, Vol.4, pp. 87-90.

[5] Alday, L.; Bruno, E.; Moreyra, E.; et al. (1998). Mid term results of dual-chamber pacing in children with hypertrophic obstructive cardiomyopathy. *Echocardiography*, Vol.15, pp. 289-295.

[6] Alday, L.; Moreyra, E.; Bruno, E.; et al. (2010). Left ventricular noncompaction associated with hypertrophic cardiomyopathy and Wolff-Parkinson-White syndrome. *Health*, Vol.2, pp. 200-3.

[7] Aoun, N.; Fernandes, L.; Succi, E.; et al. (1994). Beta-hemolytic streptococcus endocarditis in an adolescent with hypertrophic cardiomyopathy. *Arq Bras Cardiol*, Vol.63, pp. 211-3.

[8] Arad, M.; Maron, B.; Gorham, J.; et al. (2005). Glycogen storage diseases presenting as hypertrophic cardiomyopathy. *N Eng J Med*, Vol.352, pp. 362-72.

[9] Basso, C.; Thiene, G.; Corrado, D.; et al. (2000). Hypertrophic cardiomyopathy and sudden death in the young: pathologic evidence of myocardial ischemia. *Hum Pathol*, Vol.31, pp. 988-98.

[10] Berger, S.; Dhala, A. & Dearani J. (2009). State-of-the-art management of hypertrophic cardiomyopathy in children. *Cardiol Young*, Vol.19 (suppl 2), pp. 66-73.

[11] Berul, C.; Van Hare, G., Kertesz, N.; et al. (2008). Results of a multicenter retrospective implantable cardioverter-defibrillator registry of pediatric and congenital heart disease patients. *J Am Coll Cardiol* Vol.51, 1685-91.

[12] Biagini, E.; Coccolo, F.; Ferlito, M.; et al. (2005) Dilated-hypokinetic evolution of hypertrophic cardiomyopathy. Prevalence, incidence, risk factors, and prognostic implications in pediatric and adult patients. *J Am Coll Cardiol, Vol.* 46: 1543-50.

[13] Bobkowski, W.; Sobieszczańska, M.; Turska-Kmieć, A.; et al. (2007). Mutation of the MYH7 gene in a child with hypertrophic cardiomyopathy and Wolff-Parkinson-White syndrome. *J Appl Genet*, Vol.48, pp. 185-8.

[14] Bos, J.; Towbin, J. & Ackerman, M. (2009). Diagnostic, prognostic, and therapeutic implications of genetic testing for hypertrophic cardiomyopathy. *J Am Coll Cardiol*, Vol.54, pp. 201-11.

[15] Braunwald, E.; Lambrew, C.; Rockoff, S.; et al. (1964). Idiopathic hypertrophic subaortic stenosis. I. A description of the disease based upon an analysis of 64 patients. *Circulation*, Vol.30 (suppl. IV), pp. 3-119.

[16] Brock, R. & Fleming, P. (1956). Aortic subvalvar stenosis. *Guys Hosp Rep*, Vol.105: pp. 391-408.

[17] Bruder, O.; Wagner, A.; Jensen, C.; et al. (2010). Myocardial scar visualized by cardiovascular magnetic resonance imaging predicts major adverse events in patients with hypertrophic cardiomyopathy. *J Am Coll Cardiol*, Vol,56, pp. 875-87.

[18] Bruno, E.; Maisuls, H.; Juaneda, E.; et al. (2002). Clinical features of hypertrophic cardiomyopathy in the young. *Cardiol Young*, Vol.12, pp. 147-52.

[19] Burch, M.; Mann, J.; Sharland, M.; et al. (1992). Myocardial disarray in Noonan syndrome. *Br Heart J*, Vol.68, pp. 586-8.

[20] Cardim, N.; Oliveira, A.; Longo, S.; et al. (2003). Doppler tissue imaging: regional myocardial function in hypertrophic cardiomyopathy and in athlete's heart. *J Am Soc Echocardiogr*, Vol.16, pp. 223-32.

[21] Chimenti, C.; Pieroni, M.; Morgante, E.; et al. (2004). Prevalence of Fabry disease in female patients with late-onset hypertrophic cardiomyopathy. *Circulation*, Vol.110, pp. 1047-53.

[22] Colan, S.; Lipshultz, S.; Lowe, A.; et al. (2007). Epidemiology and cause-specific outcome of hypertrophic cardiomyopathy in children. Findings from the Pediatric Cardiomyopathy Registry. *Circulation*, Vol.115, pp. 773-81.

[23] Denfield, S.; Rosenthal, G.; Gajarski, R.; et al. (1997). Restrictive cardiomyopathies in childhood. Etiologies and natural histories. *Tex Heart Inst J*, Vol.24, pp.38-44.

[24] Decker, J.; Rossano, J.; O'Brian Smith, E.; et al. (2009). Risk factors and mode of death in isolated hypertrophic cardiomyopathy in children. *J Am Coll Cardiol*, Vol.54, pp. 250-4.

[25] Ehlers, J.; Hagstrom, J.; Lukas, D.; et al. (1962). Glycogen storage disease of the myocardium with obstruction to left ventricular outflow. *Circulation*, Vol.25, pp.96-109.

[26] Eidem, B.; Jones, C. & Cetta, F. (2000). Unusual association of hypertrophic cardiomyopathy with complete atrioventricular canal defect and Down syndrome. *Tex Heart Inst J*, Vol.27, pp. 289-91.

[27] Elliott, P.; Poloniecki, J.; Dickie, S.; et al. (2000). Sudden death in hypertrophic cardiomyopathy: identification of high risk patients. *J Am Coll Cardiol*, Vol.36, pp. 2212-8.

[28] Elliott, P.; Andersson, B.; Arbustini, E.; et al. (2008). Classification of the cardiomyopathies: a position statement from the European Society of Cardiology Working Group on Myocardial and Pericardial Diseases. *Eur Heart J*, Vol .29(2), pp. 270-6.

[29] Eng, C.; Guffon, N.; Wilcox, W.; et al. (2001). Safety and efficacy of recombinant human alpha-galactosidase. A replacement therapy in Fabry's disease. *N Eng J Med*, Vol.345, pp. 9-16.

[30] Epstein, A.; Dimarco, J.; Ellenbogen, K.; et al. (2008). ACC/AHA/HRS 2008 guidelines for device-based therapy of cardiac rhythm abnormalities. *Heart Rhythm*, Vol.5, pp. e1-62.

[31] Falicov, R.; Resnekov, L. (1977). Mid ventricular obstruction in hypertrophic obstructive cardiomyopathy. New diagnostic and therapeutic challenge. *Brit Heart J*, Vol.39, pp. 701-5.

[32] Fananapazir, L.; Cannon, R.; Tripodi, D.; et al. (1992). Impact of dual chamber permanent pacing in patients with obstructive hypertrophic cardiomyopathy with symptoms refractory to verapamil and beta adrenergic blocker therapy. *Circulation*, Vol.85, pp. 2149-61.

[33] Ferrans, V.; Morrow, A.; Roberts, W. (1972). Myocardial ultrastructure in idiopathic hypertrophic subaortic stenosis: a study of operatively excised left ventricular outflow tract muscle in 14 patients. *Circulation*, Vol.45, pp. 769-92

[34] Franklin, R., Anderson, R., Elliot, M., et al. (1999). The European pediatric cardiac code. *Cardiol Young*, Vol.9, pp. 633-57.

[35] Galve, E.; Sambola, A.; Saldaña, G.; et al. (2010). Late benefits of dual-chamber pacing in obstructive hypertrophic cardiomyopathy: a 10-year follow-up study. *Heart*, Vol .96, pp. 352-6.

[36] Gottdiener, J.; Hawley, R.; Maron, B.; et al. (1982). Characteristics of the cardiac hypertrophy in Friedreich's ataxia. *Am Heart J*, Vol.103, pp. 525-31.

[37] Gregor, P.; Widimsky, P.; Cenenka, V; et al. (1989). Electrocardiographic changes can precede the development of myocardial hypertrophy in the setting of hypertrophic cardiomyopathy. *Int J Cardiol*, Vol.23, pp. 335-41.

[38] Grenier, M.; Osganian, S.; Cox, G.; et al. (2000). Design and implementation of the North American Pediatric Cardiomyopathy Registry. *Am Heart J*, Vol.139, pp. 586-95.

[39] Grigg, L.; Wigle, E.; Williams, W.; et al. (1992). Transesophageal Doppler echocardiography in obstructive hypertrophic cardiomyopathy: classification of pathophysiology and importance in intraoperative decision making. *J Am Coll Cardiol*, Vol.20, pp. 42-52.

[40] Gruner, C.; Care, M.; Siminovitch, K.; et al. (2011). Sarcomere protein gene mutations in patients with apical hypertrophic cardiomyopathy. *Circ Cardiovasc Genet*, Vol.4, pp. 288-95.

[41] Harris, K.; Spirito, P.; Maron, M.; et al. (2006). Prevalence, clinical profile, and significance of left ventricular remodeling in the end-stage phase of hypertrophic cardiomyopathy. *Circulation*, Vol.114, pp. 216-25.

[42] Henry,W. ; Clark, C. & Epstein, S. (1973). Asymmetric septal hypertrophy (ASH): a unifyimg link in the IHSS disease spectrum. Observations regarding its pathogenesis, pathophysiology, and course. *Circulation*, Vol.47, pp. 827-32.

[43] Hers, H. (1963). Alpha-glucosidase deficiency in generalizad glycogen storage disease (Pompe's disease). *Biochem J*, Vol.86, pp. 11-6.

[44] Ho, C.; Lopez, B.; Coelho-Filho, O; et al. (2010). Myocardial fibrosis as an early manifestation of hyprtrophic cardiomyopathy. *New Eng J Med*, Vol.363, pp. 552-63.

[45] Jensen, M.; Almaas, V.; Jacobsson, L.; et al. (2011) Long-term outcome of percutaneous transluminal septal myocardial ablation in hypertrophic obstructive cardiomyopathy. A Scandinavian multicenter study. *Circ Cardiovasc Interv*, Vol.4, pp. 256-265.

[46] Kaski, J.; Syrris, P.; Esteban, M.; et al. (2009). Prevalence of sarcomere protein gene mutations in preadolescent children with hypertrophic cardiomyopathy. *Circ Cardiovasc Genet*, Vol.2, pp. 436-41.

[47] Kawai, C.; Kato, S.; Takashima, M.; et al. (2000). Heart disease in Friedreich's ataxia: observation of a case for half a century. *Jpn Circ J*, Vol.64, pp. 229-36.

[48] Kim, L.; Devereux, R. & Basson, C. (2011). Impact of genetic insight into Mendelian disease on cardiovascular clinical practice. *Circulation*, Vol.123, pp. 544-50.

[49] Kishnani, P.; Austin, S.; Arn, P.; et al. (2010) Glycogen storage disease type III diagnosis and management guidelines. *Genet Med*, Vol.12, pp.446-63.

[50] Klues, H.; Maron, B.; Dollar, A.; et al. (1992) Diversity of structural mitral valve alterations in hypertrophyc cardiomyopathy. *Circulation*, Vol.85, pp. 1651-60.

[51] Kuhl, H. & Hanrath P. (2004). The impact of transesophageal echocardiography on daily clinical practice. *Eur J Echocardiogr*, Vol.5, pp. 455-68.

[52] Lipshultz, S.; Sleeper, L.; Towbin, J.; et al. (2003). The incidence of pediatric cardiomyopathy in two regions of the United States. *New Eng J Med*, Vol.348, pp. 1647-55.

[53] Louie, E. & Maron, B. (1987). Apical hypertrophic cardiomyopathy: clinical and two dimensional echocardiographic assessment. *Ann Intern Med*, Vol.106, pp. 663-70.

[54] Marian A.J. (2007). Hypertrophic cardiomyopathy, in *Cardiovascular genetics and genomics for the cardiologist,* Dzau & Liew, pp. 30-54, Blackwell Futura ISBN: 978-1-4051-3394-4, Malden, Massachusetts.

[55] Maron, B. ; Roberts, W.; & Epstein, S. (1982). Sudden death in hypertrophic cardiomyopathy : a profile of 78 patients. *Circulation,* Vol.65, pp. 1388-94.

[56] Maron, B.; Spirito, P.; Wesley, Y.; et al. (1986). Development and progression of left ventricular hypertrophy in children with hypertrophic cardiomyopathy. *New Engl J Med,* Vol.315, pp. 610-4.

[57] Maron, B.; Pelliccia, A.; Spataro, A.; et al. (1993). Reduction in left ventricular wall thickness after decondinioning in highly trained Olimpic athletes. *Br Heart J,* Vol.69; pp. 125-128.

[58] Maron, B.; Gardin, J.; Flack, J.; et al. (1995a). Prevalence of hypertrophic cardiomyopathy in a general population of young adults: echocardiographic analysis of 4111 subjects in the CARDIA Study Coronary Artery Risk Development in (Young) Adults. *Circulation,* Vol.92, pp. 785-89.

[59] Maron, B.; Pelliccia, A. & Spirito, P. (1995b). Cardiac disease in young trained athletes: insights into methods for distinguishing athlete's heart from structural heart disease with particular emphasis on hypertrophic cardiomyopathy. *Circulation,* Vol.91, pp. 1596-1601.

[60] Maron, B.; Olivotto, I.; Spirito, P.; et al. (2000a). Epidemiology of hypertrophic cardiomyopathy-related death: revisited in a large non-referral-based patient population. *Circulation,* Vol.102, pp. 858-64.

[61] Maron, B.; Shen, W-K.; Links, M.; et al. (2000b). Efficacy of implantable cardioverter-defibrillators for the prevention of sudden death in patients with hypertrophic cardiomyopathy. *N Engl J Med,* Vol.342, pp. 365-73.

[62] Maron, B., McKenna, W., Danielson, G., et al. (2003a). American College of Cardiology/European Society of Cardiology clinical expert consensus document on hypertrophic cardiomyopathy. *J Am Coll Cardiol,* Vol.42, pp. 1687-713.

[63] Maron, B.; Estes, N., III; Maron, M.; et al. (2003b). Primary prevention of sudden death as a novel treatment strategy in hypertrophic cardiomyopathy. *Circulation,* Vol.107, pp. 2872-75.

[64] Maron, B.; Seidman, J. & Seidman, C. (2004). Proposal for contemporary screening strategies in families with hypertrophic cardiomyopathy. *J Am Coll Cardiol,* Vol.44, pp. 2125-32.

[65] Maron, B., Towbin, J., Thiene, G., et al. (2006). Contemporary definitions and classification of the cardiomyopathies. *Circulation,* Vol.113, pp. 1807-16.

[66] Maron, B.; Maron, M.; Wigle, E.; et al. (2009). The 50-year history, controversy, and clinical implications of left ventricular outflow tract obstruction in hypertrophic cardiomyopathy. *J Am Coll Cardiol,* Vol. 54 (3), pp. 191-200.

[67] Maron, M.; Olivotto, J.; Bettochi, S.; et al. (2003). Effect of left ventricular outflow tract obstruction on clinical outcome in hypertrophic obstructive cardiomyopathy. *New Eng J Med,* Vol.348, pp. 295-303.

[68] Maron, M.; Olivotto, I.; Zenovich, A.; et al. (2006). Hypertrophic cardiomyopathy is predominantly a disease of left ventricular outflow tract obstruction. *Circulation,* Vol.114, pp. 2232-9.

[69] Maron, M.; Appelbaum, E.; Harrigan, C.; et al. (2008). Clinical profile and significance of delayed enhancement in hypertrophic cardiomyopathy. *Circ Heart Fail,* Vol.1, pp. 184-91.

[70] Maron, M.; Maron, B.; Harrigan, C.; et al. (2009). Hypertrophic cardiomyopathy phenotype revisited after 50 years with cardiovascular magnetic resonance. *J Am Coll Cardiol,* Vol.54, pp. 220-8.

[71] Maron, M.; Olivotto, I.; Harrigan, C.; et al. (2011). Mitral valve abnormalities identified by cardiovascular magnetic resonance represent a primary phenotypic expression of hypertrophic cardiomyopathy. *Circulation,* Vol.124, pp. 40-7.

[72] McKenna, W. & Deanfield, J. (1984). Hypertrophic cardiomyopathy. An important cause of sudden death. *Arch Dis Childhood,* Vol.59, pp. 971-75.

[73] McKenna, W.; Oakley, C.; Krikler D.; et al. (1985). Improved survival with amiodarone in patients with hypertrophic cardiomyopathy and ventricular tachycardia. *Br Heart J,* Vol.53, pp. 412-6.

[74] McKenna, W.; Franklin, R.; Nihoyannopoulos, P.; et al. (1988). Arrhythmia and prognosis in infants, children and adolescents with hypertrophic cardiomyopathy. *J Am Coll Cardiol,* Vol.11, pp. 147-53.

[75] McMahon, C.; Nagueh, S.; Pignatelli, R.; et al. (2004). Characterization of left ventricular diastolic function by tissue Doppler imaging and clinical status in children with hypertrophic cardiomyopathy. *Circulation,* Vol.109, pp. 1756-62.

[76] Michael, S.; Petrocine, S.; Qian, J.; et al. (2006). Iron and iron-responding proteins in the cardiomyopathy of Friedreich's ataxia. *Cerebellum,* Vol.5, pp. 257-67.

[77] Minakata K.; Dearani J.; O'Leary, P,; et al. (2005). Septal myectomy for obstructive hypertrophic cardiomyopathy in pediatric patients: early and late results. *Ann Thorac Surg,* Vol.80, pp. 1424-30.

[78] Minami, Y.; Kajimoto, K.; Terajima, Y.; et al. (2011). Clinical implications of midventricular obstruction in patients with hypertrophic cardiomyopathy. *J Am Coll Cardiol,* Vol.57, pp. 2346-55.

[79] Moolman, J.; Corfield, V.; Posen, B.; et al. (1997). Sudden death due to troponin T mutations. *J Am Coll Cardiol,* Vol.29, pp. 549-55.

[80] Moreyra, E.; Buteler, B.; Madoery, R.; et al. (1972) Drugs and maneuvers in the diagnosis of muscular subaortic stenosis. *Am Heart J,* Vol.83, pp. 431-3.

[81] Morgan-Hughes, G. & Motwani, J. (2002). Mitral valve endocarditis in hypertrophic cardiomyopathy: case report and literature review. *Heart,* Vol.87, pp. e8.

[82] Nagueh, S.; McFalls, J.; Meyer, D.; et al. (2003). Tissue Doppler imaging predicts the development of hypertrophic cardiomyopathy in subjects with subclinical disease. *Circulation,* Vol.108, pp. 395-8.

[83] Noonan, J. (1968). Hypertelorysm with Turner phenotype: a new syndrome with associated congenital heart disease. *Am J Dis Child,* Vol.116, pp. 373-80.

[84] Nora, J.; Nora, A.; Sinha, A.; et al. (1974). The Ulrich-Noonan syndrome (Turner phenotype). *Am J Dis Child,* Vol.127, pp. 48-55.

[85] Nora, J.; Lortscher, R. & Spangler, R. (1975). Echocardiographic studies of left ventricular disease in Ulrich-Noonan syndrome. *Am J Dis Child,* Vol.129, pp. 1417-20.

[86] Nugent, A.; Daubeney, P.; Chondros, P.; et al. (2003). The epidemiology of childhood cardiomyopathy in Australia. *New Eng J Med,* Vol.348, pp. 1703-5.

[87] Nugent, A.; Daubeney, P.; Chondros, P.; et al. (2005). Clinical features and outcomes of childhood hypertrophic cardiomyopathy. Results from a national population-based study. *Circulation*, Vol.112, pp. 1332-8.

[88] Niimura, H.; Bachinski, L.; Sangwatanaroj, S.; et al. (1998). Mutations in the gene for cardiac myosin-binding protein C and late-onset familial hypertrophic cardiomyopathy. *N Eng J Med*, Vol.338, pp. 1248-57.

[89] Ostman-Smith, I.; Wettrell, G.; Keeton, B.; et al. (2005). Echocardiographic and electrocardiographic identification of those children with hypertrophic cardiomyopathy who should be considered at high-risk of dying suddenly. *Cardiol Young*, Vol.15, pp. 632-42.

[90] Panza, J. & Maron, B. (1989). Relation of electrocardiographic abnormalities to evolving left ventricular hypertrophy in hypertrophic cardiomyopathy during childhood. *Am J Cardiol*, Vol.63, pp. 1258-65.

[91] Panza, J.; Maris, T. & Maron, B. (1992). Development and determinants of dynamic obstruction to left ventricular outflow in young patients with hypertrophic cardiomyopathy. *Circulation*, Vol.85, pp. 1398-405.

[92] Peirone, A.; Bruno, E.; Rossi, N.; et al. (2005). Woolly hair and palmoplantar hyperkeratosis may present with hypertrophic cardiomyopathy. *Pediatr Cardiol*, Vol.26, pp. 470-2.

[93] Roberts, A.; Allanson, J.; Jadico, S.; et al. (2006). The cardiofaciocutaneous syndrome. *J Med Genet*, Vol.43, pp. 833-842.

[94] Rosen, K.; Cameron, R.; Bigham, P. (1997). Hypertrophic cardiomyopathy presenting with 3rd-degree atrioventricular block. *Texas Heart J*, Vol.24, pp. 372-5.

[95] Sachdev, B.; Takenaka, T.; Teraguchi, H.; et al. (2002). Prevalence of Anderson-Fabry disease in male patients with late onset hypertrophic cardiomyopathy. *Circulation*, Vol.105, pp. 1407-11.

[96] Seidman, J. & Seidman, C. (2001). The genetic basis for cardiomyopathy: from mutation identification to mechanistic paradigms. *Cell*, Vol.104, pp. 557-67.

[97] Seidman, C. & Seidman, J. (2011). Identifying sarcomere gene mutations in hypertrophic cardiomyopathy. *Circ Res*. Vol.108, pp. 743-50.

[98] Shah, P.; Gramiak, R. & Kramer, D. (1969). Ultrasound localization of left ventricular outflow obstruction in hypertrophic obstructive cardiomyopathy. *Circulation*, Vol.40, pp. 3-11.

[99] Shah, P.; Gramiak, R.; Adelman, A.; et al. (1971). Role of echocardiography in diagnostic and hemodynamic assessment of hypertrophic subaortic stenosis. *Circulation*, Vol.44, pp. 891-8.

[100] Sherrid, M.; Chu, C.; Delia, E.; et al. (1993). An echocardiographic study of the fluid mechanics of obstruction in hypertrophic cardiomyopathy. *J Am Coll Cardiol*, Vol.22, pp. 816-25.

[101] Sherrid, M.; Barac, I.; McKenna, W.; et al. (2005). Multicenter study of the efficacy and safety of disopyramide in obstructive hypertrophic cardiomyopathy. *J Am Coll Cardiol*, Vol.45, pp. 1251-8.

[102] Shirani, J.; Maron, B.; Cannon, R.; et al. (1993). Clinicopathologic features of hypertrophic cardiomyopathy managed by cardiac transplantation. *Am J Cardio*, Vol.72, pp.434-40.

[103] Sigwart, U. (1995). Non-surgical myocardial reduction for hypertrophic obstructive cardiomyopathy. *Lancet*, Vol.346, pp. 211-4.

[104] Somerville, J. & Becu, L. (1978). Congenital heart disease associated with hypertrophic cardiomyopathy. *Br Heart J*, Vol.40, pp. 1034-39.

[105] Sznajer, Y.; Keren, B.; Baumann, C.; et al. (2007). The spectrum of cardiac anomalies in Noonan syndrome as a result of mutations in the *PTPN11* gene. *Pediatrics*, Vol.119, pp. e1325-31.

[106] Tartaglia, M.; Mehler, E.; Goldberg, R.; et al. (2001). Mutations in PTPN11, encoding the protein tyrosine phosphatase SHP-2, cause Noonan syndrome. *Nat Genet*, Vol.29, pp. 465-8.

[107] Teare, D. (1958). Asymmetrical hypertrophy of the heart in young adults. *Br Heart J*, Vol.20, pp. 1-8.

[108] Tikanoja, T.; Jaaskelainen, P.; Laakso, M.; et al. (1999). Simultaneous hypertrophic cardiomyopathy and ventricular septal defect in children. *Am J Cardiol*, Vol.84, pp. 485-6.

[109] Watkins, H.; Rosenzweig, A.; Hwang, D.; et al. (2009). Characteristic and prognostic implications of myosin missense mutations in familial hypertrophic cardiomyopathy. *N Eng J Med*, Vol.326, pp. 1108-14.

[110] Wigle, E.; Auger, P. & Marquis, Y. (1967). Muscular subaortic stenosis. The direct relation between the intraventricular pressure difference and the left ventricular ejection time. *Circulation*, Vol.36, pp. 36-44.

[111] Winkel, L.; Hagemans, M.; van Doorn, P.; et al. (2005). The natural course of non-classic Pompe's disease; a review of 225 published cases. *J Neurol*, Vol.252, pp. 875-84.

[112] Yamaguchi, H.; Ishimura, T.; Nishiyama, S.; et al. (1979). Hypertrophic nonobstructive cardiomyopathy with giant negative T waves (apical hypertrophy): ventriculographic and echocardiographic features in 30 patients. *Am J Cardiol*, Vol.44, pp. 401-12.

7

Quality of Life in Dilated Cardiomyopathy with Refractory Chronic Heart Failure Undergoing Devices Implantation

Elisabete Nave Leal[1], José Luís Pais Ribeiro[2] and Mário Martins Oliveira[3]
[1]Polytechnic Institute of Lisbon /School of Health Technology of Lisbon
[2]University of Porto/Faculty of Psychology and Educational Sciences
[3]Lisbon Central Hospital Center, Santa Marta Hospital
Portugal

1. Introduction

Heart failure is the final stage of most of cardiac diseases. It is a complex syndrome in which the patients should have the following features: symptoms of heart failure, typically shortness of breath at rest or during exertion, and/or fatigue; signs of fluid retention such as pulmonary congestion or ankle swelling; and objective evidence of an abnormality of the structure or function of the heart at rest. This progressive syndrome as a high incidence and prevalence and poor prognosis: four-year mortality is around 50% with 40% of the patients admitted to hospital dying or readmitted within a year (European Society of Cardiology, 2008). With ageing, many patients will develop chronic heart failure, which, because of its symptoms, patient's awareness of their risk of dying, and the effects of therapy, together with frequent hospitalizations, has considerable impact on patient's health-related quality of life.

In the actual field of management, implantable devices have an important role for select patients. According to the European Society of Cardiology guidelines for the diagnosis and treatment of acute and chronic heart failure (2008), cardiac resynchronization therapy with defibrillator function is recommended to reduce morbidity and mortality in patients in New York Heart Association III-IV class who are symptomatic despite optimal medical therapy, and who have a reduced ejection fraction (left ventricular ejection fraction ≤35%) and QRS prolongation (QRS width ≥120 ms) and implantable cardioverter-defibrillator is recommended for primary prevention of sudden death to reduce mortality in patients with ventricular dysfunction due to prior myocardial infarction or non-ischemic cardiomyopathy with a left ventricular ejection fraction ≤35% in New York Heart Association functional class II or III, receiving optimal medical therapy, and who have reasonable expectation of survival with good functional status for more than one year.

The effect of these therapies in the quality of life in general and regarding the type of therapeutic response in particular is a field under investigation.

The aim of this study was to evaluate the impact of cardiac resynchronization therapy and implantable cardioverter-defibrillator in the quality of life of patients with chronic heart failure refractory to optimal pharmacological therapy in the first six months after device implantation.

2. Method

2.1 Participants

From ninety-six patients with chronic heart failure refractory to optimal pharmacological therapy in consecutive sequential analysis, fifty-two underwent implantation of cardiac resynchronization therapy system combined with implantable cardioverter-defibrillator and forty-four systems with implantable cardioverter-defibrillator alone for primary prevention of sudden death.

In the cardiac resynchronization therapy group, age was 64,2±8,9 (37-78) years with 35 males and 17 females, left ventricular ejection fraction was 24,6±5,4 (11-35)% and 94% in class III of the New York Heart Association classification. The etiology was mostly idiopathic (46,2%) or ischemic (34,6%).

In the implantable cardioverter-defibrillator group, age was 61,1±12,6 (25-83) years with 38 males and 6 females, left ventricular ejection fraction was 26,1±5,4 (15-37)% and 82,9% in class II of New York Heart Association classification. The etiology was mostly ischemic (75%) (Figure 1).

	Characteristics	Cardiac Resyncrhronization Therapy	Implantable Cardioverter-Defibrillator
Age	M	64,2	61,1
	DP	8,9	12,6
Gender	Male	67,3%	86,4%
	Female	32,7%	13,6%
Left Ventricular Ejection Fraction	M	24,6%	26,1%
	DP	5,4	5,4
New York Heart Association Classification	Class I	0%	0%
	Class II	4,0%	82,9%
	Class III	94%	17,1%
	Class IV	2%	0%
Etiology of Chronic Heart Failure	Ischemic	34,6%	75,0%
	Hypertensive	7,7%	0%
	Valvular	7,7%	2,3%
	Idiopathic	46,2%	20,5%
	Other	3,8%	2,3%

Fig. 1. Population Characteristics

2.2 Instruments and procedure

Patients were assessed at admission, immediately before the intervention, and in the outpatient clinic within 6 months. We considered functionality by the New York Heart Association classification, left ventricular ejection fraction and the quality of life Kansas City Cardiomyophathy Questionnaire.

The Kansas City Cardiomyopathy Questionnaire (Green et al., 2000) validated for the portuguese population (Nave-Leal et al., 2010) is composed of twenty three items divided into five domains: physical limitation, symptoms, quality of life, self-efficacy and social interference. The physical limitation domain measures the extent to which congestive heart failure symptoms have limited some of the patient's physical activities over the previous two weeks. The symptom domain assesses the number of times that congestive heart failure symptoms such as fatigue, dyspnea or limb edema have occurred in the previous two weeks and whether there have been changes in symptoms during the same period. The self-efficacy domain measures the patient's knowledge of how to avoid worsening of symptoms and of what to do if this occurs. The quality of life domain evaluates patients' perception of their enjoyment of life and of their sense of discouragement due to their heart failure, while the social interference domain assesses how congestive heart failure affects the patient's lifestyle. To facilitate interpretability, two summary scores were developed: the first, the functional status score, combines the physical limitation and symptom domains, and the second, the clinical summary score, combines the functional status score with the quality of life and social interference domains (Figure 2).

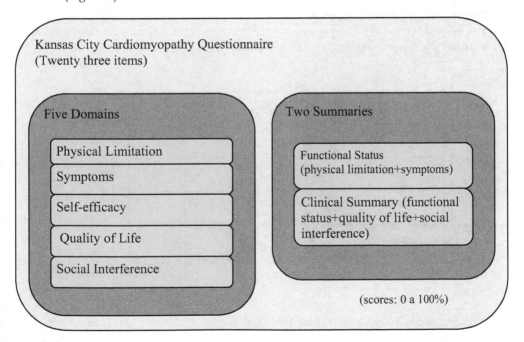

Fig. 2. Domains and Summaries of the Kansas City Cardiomyopathy Questionnaire

His psychometrics proprieties shows that it's a good instrument regarding fidelity, validity, sensitive to clinical change and specific to measure quality of life in a population with chronic heart failure.

The New York Heart Association classification (The Criteria Committee of the New York Heart Association, 1994 cited by European Society of Cardiology, 2008) measures the functional capacity based on the severity of symptoms and limitation of physical activity and is the most widely used measure to assess functionality of cardiac patients. Class I is defined as the absence of limitations on the exercise usually does not cause fatigue, dyspnoea or palpitations; Class II is characterized by a slight limitation of physical activity, being comfortable at rest but ordinary physical activity causes fatigue, palpitations or dyspnea; Class III is defined by a marked limitation of physical activity, being comfortable at rest but in a less intense activity that usually causes symptoms of heart failure, class IV is characterized by an inability to perform any physical activity without discomfort, where the symptoms of heart failure are present.

The left ventricular ejection fraction calculated by echocardiography in a percentage below 35% is indicative of poor prognosis.

3. Results

During the first six months of follow-up post-implant there was no detection of sustained ventricular tachyarrhythmias.

3.1 Cardiac resynchronization therapy

Cardiac resynchronization therapy was associated with improved functionality with New York Heart Association classification, from 3,0±0,2 to 2,1±0,5, $p<0.05$ (Figure 3).

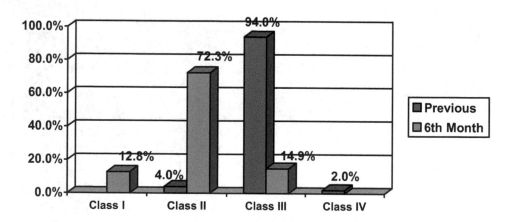

Fig. 3. Functionality at 6th Month Follow-up in Cardiac Resynchronization Therapy

This therapy improved left ventricular ejection fraction, from 24,6±6,4% to 35,5±11,9%, $p<0.05$ (Figure 4).

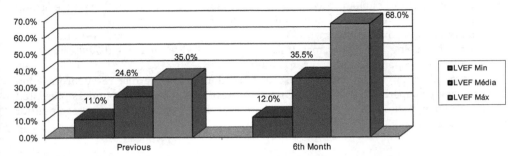

Fig. 4. Left Ventricular Ejection Fraction (LVEF) at 6th Month Follow-up in Cardiac Resynchronization Therapy

Cardiac resynchronization therapy improved quality of life in the various fields and sums assessed except for the self-efficacy domain, high before this therapy (from 81,6±28,9 to 88,1±24,1, non significant): physical limitation domain from 52,3±26,7 to 83,1±23,6; symptoms domain from 55,6±27,6 to 80,1±22,3; quality of life domain from 37,4±30,1 to 75,9±28,6; social interference domain from 57,8±30,9 to 84,6±25,9; functional status sum from 55,7±25,6 to 82,7±20,7 and clinical summary sum from 53,1±25,7 to 81,1±22,1,$\rho<0.05$ (Figure 5).

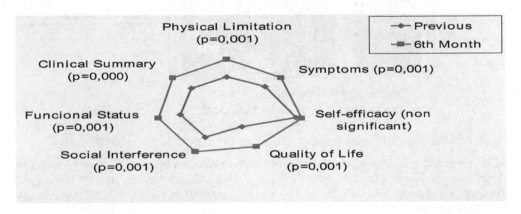

Fig. 5. Quality of Life at 6th Month Follow-up in Cardiac Resynchronization Therapy

We have stratified some of these patients regarding the type of therapeutic response: thirty four patients responded to this therapeutic and nine did not respond to cardiac resynchronization therapy.

Fifteen patients have a left ventricular ejection fraction superior to 45% post cardiac resynchronization therapy and were classified as super-responders, nineteen patients have a sustained improvement in functional class and an increase in left ventricular ejection fraction of 15% and were classified as responders and nine patients have no clinical or left ventricular ejection fraction improvement and were classified as non-responders.

The age and the etiology was identical (65,1±8,2 years between 48-75 years, 63,2±11,1 years between 37-78 and 62,8±6,1 years between 55-71 years for super-responders, responders e non-responders respectively and etiology mainly idiopathic with the majority of the cases followed by ischemic etiology according to the results described for the whole group submitted to cardiac resynchronization therapy) but the gender was different with super-responders being in majority women (53,3% female and 46,7% male) and responders and non responders being in majority men (84,2% male and 15,8% female and 77,8% men and 22,2% female for responders and non-responders respectively).

Super-responders had a left ventricular ejection fraction prior to cardiac resynchronization therapy average superior to 25% (29,5±4,5) while responders and non responders presented a left ventricular ejection fraction prior to cardiac resynchronization therapy average inferior to 25% (22,6±6,2 and 23,9±6,5) (Figure 6).

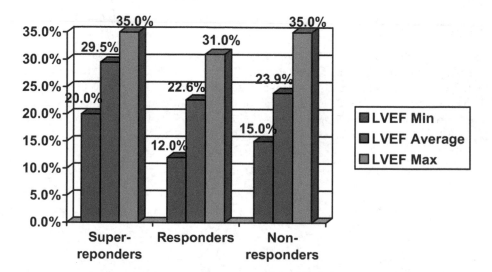

Fig. 6. Left Ventricular Ejection Fraction Regarding the Type of Therapeutic Response

Super responders and responder had the all of their patients in class III of the New York Heart Association classification prior to therapy while non-responders despite having the majority of the patients in class III (66,7%) also had patients in class II (22,2%) and class IV (11,1%) of the New York Heart Association classification prior to therapy (Figure 7).

Non responders presented a low quality of life before this therapy and have not perceived any improvement on their quality of life (physical limitation domain from 25,2±21,9 to 59,1±37,4; symptoms domain from 46,5±33,3 to 63,6±28,2; self-efficacy domain from 95,8±7,3 to 97,59±7,1; quality of life domain from 20,8±27,4 to 52,1±35,1; social interference domain from 37,5±31,5 to 63,8±36,8; functional status sum from 38,1±28,9 to 63,8±30,4 and clinical summary sum from 34,8±28,4 to 60,1±32,2) (Figure 8).

Super-responders and responders started with a better perception of their quality of life and identify improvement in quality of life in all dimensions and sums,p≤0,05 except for the auto-efficacy dimension in responders where there was no statistical significant change (physical limitation domain from 51,8±24,6 to 90,4,1±13,7; symptoms domain from 53,9±27,6 to 84,5±21,8; self-efficacy domain from 76,2±34,3 to 95,7±11,6; quality of life domain from 38,7±31,6 to 85,1±24,5; social interference domain from 55,8±27,1 to 85,7±28,9; functional status sum from 55,3±22,6 to 87,7±17,4 and clinical summary sum from 52,6±23,4 to

60,1±32,2 for super responders and physical limitation domain from 63,1±23,7 to 89,1±15,3; symptoms domain from 60,1±25,7 to 82,4±20,9; self-efficacy domain from 76,9±33,1 to 83,3±26,8; quality of life domain from 39,8±27,4 to 75,1±27,6; social interference domain from 63,9±31,7 to 90,2±18,3; functional status sum from 62,6±23,8 to 86,6±15,7 and clinical summary sum from 59,2±23,7 to 84,9±17,8 for responders) (Figure 9 and Figure 10).

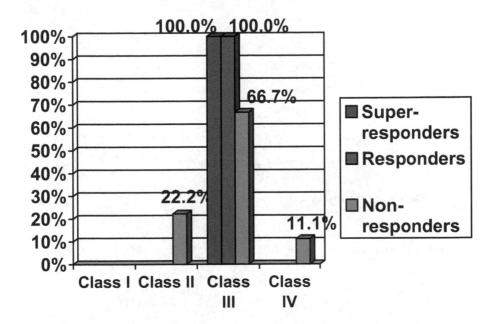

Fig. 7. New York Heart Association Classification Regarding the Type of Therapeutic Response

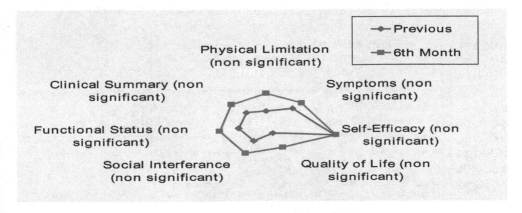

Fig. 8. Quality of Life in Non-responders

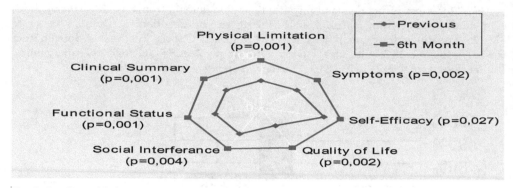

Fig. 9. Quality of Life in Super-responders

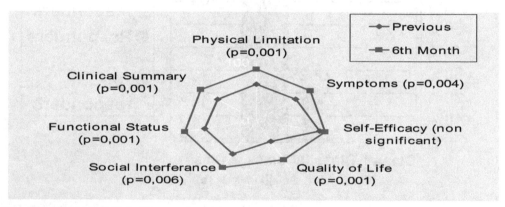

Fig. 10. Quality of Life in Responders

3.2 Implantable cardioverter-defibrillator
Implantable cardioverter defibrillator was associated with improved functionality with New York Heart Association classification from 2,1±0,3 to 1,9±0,5 $\rho<0.05$ (Figure 11).

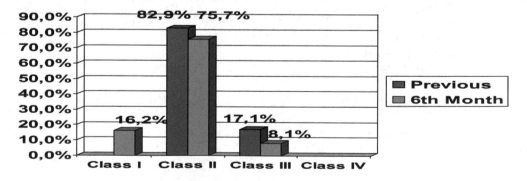

Fig. 11. Functionality at 6th Month Follow-up in Implantable Cardioverter Defibrillator

This device was not associated with improvement in left ventricular ejection fraction (from 26,1±5,4 to 26,4±5,9), where changes were no significant (Figure 12).

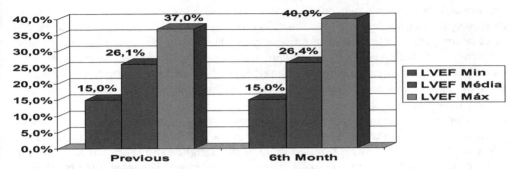

Fig. 12. Left Ventricular Ejection Fraction (LVEF) at 6th Month Follow-up in Implantable Cardioverter Defibrillator

Implantable cardioverter-defibrillator improved quality of life only in social interference domain from 73,9±34,4 to 82,7±27,5, quality of life domain from 54,3±32,1 to 71,1±28,1 and clinical summary sum from 72,4±24,1 to 78,4±25,1,p<0.05. In the physical limitation domain (from 76,2±24,5 to 80,4±26,1), symptoms domain (from 73,6±24,7 to 78,1±24,6), self-efficacy domain (from 80,3±26,2 to 83,6±25,1) and functional status sum (from 76,2±23,1 to 80,4±23,9), changes were no significant (Figure 13). Initial scores in every dimension and sum were high before the implantation of this device.

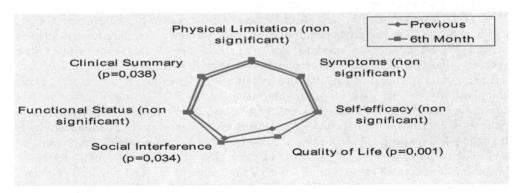

Fig. 13. Quality of Life at 6th Month Follow-up in Implantable Cardioverter Defibrillator

4. Discussion

In this study the cardiac resynchronization therapy combined with implantable cardioverter-defibrillator improved left ventricular function, functionality and quality of life at six months follow-up. According to the European Cardiac Society, 2008 the survival advantage of cardiac resynchronization therapy with implantable cardioverter-defibrillator has not been adequately addressed. However due to the documented effectiveness of implantable cardioverter-defibrillator therapy in the prevention of sudden cardiac death, the use of cardiac resynchronization therapy associated to implantable cardioverter-defibrillator is commonly preferred in clinical practice in patients satisfying cardiac resynchronization therapy criteria including an expectation of survival with good functional status for more than one year. Lousano et al., 2005 in the VENTAK CHF/CONTAK CD study followed 490 heart failure patients with indication for an implantable cardioverter-defibrillator compared antitachycardia pacing efficacy in patients with or without cardiac resynchronization therapy. These authors encountered that the efficacy of biventricular antitachycardia pacing in heart failure patients is significantly better in those with cardiac resynchronization therapy than in those without.

Other studies have identified the benefits of this therapy in mortality and morbidity of patients with heart failure. Bristow et al., 2004 in the COMPANION study analysed the effect of the cardiac resynchronization therapy in mortality and hospitalization among patients with advanced chronic heart failure and intraventricular conduction delays. 1520 patients in New York Heart Association class III or IV due to ischemic or non-ischemic cardiomyopathies and a QRS interval of at least 120 ms were randomly assigned in three groups to receive optimal pharmacologic therapy (diuretics, angiotensin-converting–enzyme inhibitors, beta-blockers and spironolactone) alone or in combination with cardiac resynchronization therapy with either a pacemaker or a pacemaker–defibrillator. These authors encountered that cardiac resynchronization therapy decreases the combined risk of death from any cause or first hospitalization and, when combined with an implantable defibrillator, significantly reduces mortality. Cleland et al., 2005 in the CARE-HF study analyzed the effects of cardiac resynchronization therapy on morbidity and mortality among patients with heart failure due to left ventricular systolic dysfunction and cardiac dyssynchrony. 813 patients with New York Heart Association class III or IV heart failure due to left ventricular systolic dysfunction and cardiac dyssynchrony who were receiving standard pharmacologic therapy were randomly assigned to receive medical therapy alone or with cardiac resynchronization. These authors encountered that cardiac resynchronization increases left ventricular ejection fraction, improve symptoms and the quality of life and reduce complications and the risk of death. McAlister et al., 2007 in a systematic review concerning the efficacy, effectiveness and safety of cardiac resynchronization therapy in patients with left ventricular systolic dysfunction in a total of 14 randomized trials involving 4420 patients, observed that cardiac resynchronization therapy improved left ventricular ejection fraction, quality of life and functionality and decreased hospitalizations and all cause mortality with a high implant rate and low lead problems during eleven months follow-up. They conclude that this therapy reduces morbidity and mortality in patients with left ventricular systolic dysfunction, prolonged QRS duration and New York Heart Association class III and IV symptoms when combined with optimal pharmacotherapy. About the sustained effect of this therapy Sutton et al., 2006 in the MIRACLE study followed 228 patients submitted to cardiac resynchronization therapy during twelve months post-implantation to determine whether reverse left ventricular remodeling and symptomatic benefit from this therapy were sustained at one year and if so, in what proportion. These authors encountered that reverse left ventricular remodeling and symptom benefit are sustained at twelve months in patients with New York Heart Association class III/IV heart failure but occur to a lesser degree in patients with ischemic versus non-ischemic etiology, according to them most likely owing to the inexorable progression of ischemic disease.

Despite the good results achieved with cardiac resynchronization therapy according to Santos et al., 2006 one third of the patients do not benefit from it. In our study, from forty-three patients, eight did not respond to this therapy. This group identified a low quality of live before implantation and did not perceive any improvement after cardiac resynchronization therapy. Also in this non-responding group we had patients in class II to IV of the New York Heart Association classification before intervention. Interestingly the super-responders were majority women and have a left ventricular ejection fraction prior to implantation superior to 25%. The response to this therapy was associated to improvement of quality of life perceived by the patients and a New York Heart Association class III classification before implantation. There are few studies regarding the predictors of response to this therapy. Quiao et al., 2011 in a study with seventy-six consecutive patients submitted to cardiac resynchronization therapy divided in to super-responders, responders and non-responders conclude that patients with a smaller left ventricle would have a better chance to become super-responders. Santos et al., 2006 in twenty-three consecutive patients with heart failure refractory to medical therapy who underwent cardiac resynchronization therapy studied regarding the type of response before and six months after the procedure evaluating clinical, electrocardiographic and echocardiography characteristics concluded that left ventricular dyssynchrony can be quantified by tissue Doppler imaging using QS (max-min) and values greater than 60 ms can identify responders to this therapy. This actual field under investigation requires more studies to determine the reasons for a percentage of these patients do not respond to cardiac resynchronization therapy including personal characteristics of the patients.

In this study implantable cardioverter-defibrillator alone was associated with improvement of functionality and quality of life already high in baseline due to the majority of the patients being in class II of the New York Heart Association classification. When looking to the various dimensions concerning the quality of life we stated that this improvement is observed in social and quality of life domains with this patients referring improvement of the perception of their enjoyment of life and of their sense of discouragement due to their heart failure and how congestive heart failure affects the patient's lifestyle at six month follow-up, emphasizing the necessity of looking to all dimensions evaluated in quality of life and not only the overall score to characterize the evolution of patients to clinical interventions. It is known the effect of this device on improving survival, however remains unclear the effect of this treatment in quality of life. Bardy et al., 2005 in the SCD-HeFT study concerning the effect of amiodarone or a conservatively programmed, shock-only implantable cardioverter-defibrillator in reducing the risk of death in patients with mild-to-moderate congestive heart failure, followed 2521 patients in class II or III with chronic stable heart failure due to ischemic or non-ischemic causes and left ventricular ejection fraction $\leq 35\%$ randomized for receiving amiodarone, implantable cardioverter-defibrillator or placebo. These authors encountered that in patients with mild-to-moderate congestive heart failure, conservatively programmed, shock-only implantable cardioverter-defibrillator significantly reduces risk of death while amiodarone shown no benefit compared with placebo; implantable cardioverter-defibrillator therapy had significant benefit in patients with New York Heart

Association class II but no significant effect in patients with class III; amiodarone had no benefit in patients with New York Heart Association class II and showed a significant reduction in survival in patients with class III compared to placebo. Noyes et al., 2009 in the MADIT-II study followed 938 patients randomized to receive an implantable cardioverter-defibrillator or medical therapy alone during thirty six months. These authors encountered that development of congestive heart failure and shocks among patients and their negative effect on quality of life may partially explain the lack of quality of life benefit from this therapy. Probst et al., 2011 have studied the psychological impact of implantable cardioverter-defibrillator on Brugada syndrome patients. 190 patients were divided in three groups: symptomatic implanted patients, asymptomatic implanted patients and asymptomatic patients without implantable cardioverter-defibrillator and were evaluated regarding the quality of life. These authors concluded that whatever the group, Brugada patients have a good quality of life with no difference between implanted and non-implanted patients. Despite the difficulties in their social and professional life regarding the tolerance of this device, patients considered implantation of cardioverter-defibrillator reassuring.

5. Conclusion

In a selected population with severe chronic heart failure, cardiac resynchronization therapy was associated with improvement in all domains of quality of life, functional class and left ventricular function. Regarding the type of response to this therapy, patients with positive clinical response and reverse remodeling, obtained a favorable impact in all dimensions of quality of life, while the group without response showed no improvement, with some differences between the responding and the non-responding patients like gender, perceived quality of life and the New York Heart association classification prior to implantation of the device that needs further investigation.

Implantable cardioverter-defibrillator benefits were restricted to the social dimension of quality of life and perception of life satisfaction, indicating that this intervention as no unfavorable impact in quality of life in the first six months after the implantation of this device in patients without detection of sustained ventricular tachyarrhythmias

6. Acknowledgements

The authors are grateful to the following bodies and staff of Hospital de Santa Marta: the Administrative Board; the Ethics Committee; cardiologists and cardiopneumologists of the arrhythmology clinic; and cardiologists of the heart failure clinic.

7. References

Bardy, G., Lee, K., Mark, D., Poole, J., Packer, D., Boineau, R., Domansky, M., Troutman, C., Anderson, J., Johnson, G., McNulty, S., Clapp-Channing, N., Davidson-Ray, L., Fraulo, E., Fishbein, D., Luceri, R., & Ip, J. (2005). Amiodarone or an implantable cardioverter-defibrillator for congestive heart failure.*The New England Journal of Medicine*, Vol.352,pp. 225-237

Bristow, M., Saxon, L., Boehmer, J., Krueger, S., Kass, D., De Marco, T., Carson, P., DiCarlo, L., DeMets, D., White, B., DeVries, D., & Feldman, A. (2004). Cardiac-Resynchronization Therapy with or without an Implantable Defibrillator in Advanced Chronic Heart Failure. *The New England Journal of Medicine,* Vol.350, No.21 (May 2004),pp. 2140-2150

Cleland, J., Daubert, J., Erdmam, E., Fremantle, N., Gras, D., Kappenberger, L., & Tavazzi, L. (2005). The Effect of Cardiac Resynchronization on Morbidity and Mortality in Heart Failure. *The New England Journal of Medicine,* Vol.325, No.15 (April 2005),pp. 1539-1549

European Society of Cardiology (2008). ESC Guidelines for the diagnosis and treatment of acute and chronic heart failure *2008. European Heart Journal,* vol. 29,pp. 2388-2442

Green, C., Porter, C., Bresnahan, D., & Spertus, J. (2000) Development and Evaluation of the Kansas City Cardiomyopathy Questionnaire: A New Health Status Measure for Heart Failure. *Journal of the American College of Cardiology,* Vol.35, No.5,pp. 1245-1255

Lousano, I., Higgins, S., Villa, J., Niazi, I., Toquero, J., Yong, P., Madrid, A., & Pulpón, L. (2005) Antitachycardia Pacing Efficacy Significantly Improves With Cardiac Resynchronization Therapy. *Revista Espanhola de Cardiology,* Vol.58, No.10,pp. 1148-1154

McAlister, F., Ezekowitz, J., Hooton, N., Vandermeer, B., Spooner, C., Dryden, D., Page, R., Hlatky, M., & Rowe, B. (2007). Cardiac Resynchronization Therapy for Patients with Left Ventricular Systolic Dysfunction: A Systematic Review. *Journal of the American Medical Association,* Vol.297, No.22,pp. 2502-2514

Nave-Leal, E., Pais-Ribeiro, J., Oliveira, M., Nogueira da Silva, J. Soares, R, Fragata, J. & Ferreira, R. (2010). Psychometric Properties of the Portuguese Version of the Kansas City Cardiomyopathy Questionnaire in Dilated Cardiomyopathy with Congestive Heart Failure. *Revista Portuguesa de Cardiologia,* Vol.29, No.3,pp. 353-372

Noyes, K., Corona, E., Veazie, P., Dick, A., Zhao, H., & Moss, A. (2009). Examination of the Effect of Implantable Cardioverter-Defibrillators on Health Related Quality of Life: Based on Results from the Multicenter Automatic Defibrillator Trial-II. *American Journal of Cardiovascular Drugs,* Vol.9, No.6,pp. 393-400

Probst, V., Plassard-Kerdon-Cuf, D., Mansourati, J., Mabo, P., Sacher, F., Fruchet, C., Babuty, D., Lande, G., Guyomarc´h, B., & Le Marec, H. (2011). The Psychological Impact of Implantable Cardioverter Defibrillator Implantation on Brugada Syndrome Patients. *Europace,* Vol.13, No.7,pp. 1034-1039

Quiao, Q., Ding, L., Hua, W., Chen, K., Wang, F., & Zhang, S. (2011). Potencial Predictors of Non-response to Cardiac Resynchronization Therapy. *Chinese Medical Journal,* Vol.124, No.9 (May 2011),pp. 1338-1441

Santos, J., Parreira, L., Madeira, J., Seixo, F., Mendes, L., Lopes, C., Venâncio, J., Lourenço, J., Caetano, F., Inês, L., & Mendes, M. (2006). Predictors of Response to Cardiac Resynchronization Therapy: Importance of Left Ventricular

Dyssynchrony. *Revista Portuguesa de Cardiologia*, Vol.25, No.6 (June 2006),pp. 569-581

Sutton, M., Plappert, T., Hilpisch, B., Abraham, W., Hayes, D., & Chinchoy, E. (2006). Sustained Reverse Left Ventricular Structural Remodling with Cardiac Resynchronization at One Year in Function of Etiology. *Circulation*, Vol.113,pp. 266-272

8

Peripartum Cardiomyopathy: A Systematic Review

Viviana Aursulesei and Mihai Dan Datcu

University of Medicine and Pharmacy "Gr. T. Popa", Iasi
Romania

1. Introduction

Peripartum cardiomyopathy (PPCM) is a rare but potentially life-threatening condition that occurs in previously healthy women during the last month of pregnancy and up to 5-6 months postpartum. The etiology and pathophysiology remain uncertain, although recent observations strongly suggest the specific role of prolactin cleavage secondary to unbalanced peri/postpartum oxidative stress. PPCM is a diagnosis of exclusion, as it shares many clinical characteristics with other forms of systolic heart failure secondary to cardiomyopathy. The heart failure management requires a multidisciplinary approach during pregnancy, considering the possible adverse effects on the fetus. After delivery, the treatment is in accordance with the current guidelines of heart failure. Some novel therapies, such as prolactin blockade, are proposed to either prevent or treat the patients with PPCM. A critical individual counseling concerning the risks of subsequent pregnancy must be considered. Because of its rare incidence, geographical differences, and heterogeneous presentation, PPCM continues to be incompletely characterized and understood. For all these reasons, PPCM remains a challenge in clinical practice, so future epidemiological trials and national registries are needed to learn more about the disease.

2. Historical perspective, definition, nomenclature

Peripartum cardiomyopathy has been described since the 19th century. In 1849, Ritchie was the first to establish a relationship between heart failure and puerperium (Ritchie, 1849). After 20 years, Virchow and Porak reported autopsy evidence of myocardial degeneration in females who died in the puerperium (Porak, 1880).

However, PPCM was not recognized as a distinctive form of cardiomyopathy until 1937, when Gouley et al. described the clinical and pathological features of seven pregnant women. The patients had severe or fatal heart failure associated with a dilated cardiomyopathy in the later months of pregnancy, which persisted after delivery, and autopsy findings of enlarged hearts with focal areas of fibrosis and necrosis, but no ischemic lesions. The authors remarked these features as atypical compared with those of other forms of myocardial failure and proposed that this heart failure was related to pregnancy and puerperium, directly or indirectly (Gouley et al., 1937). Since then, there were many reports on this form of cardiomyopathy. In 1965, Walsh et al. was the first to propose the specific period for the diagnosis, and highlighted that other conditions, which may be revealed by pregnancy, labor or postpartum period, must be excluded (Walsh et al., 1965).

In 1971, Demakis et al. described the natural history of 27 pregnant females who presented with cardiomegaly and congestive heart failure and defined the condition *peripartum cardiomyopathy* (Demakis et al., 1971). The investigators established 3 original diagnostic criteria, which were subsequently confirmed by the National Heart Lung and Blood Institute [NHLBI] and the Office of Rare Diseases of the National Institutes of Health [NIH] Workshop, and completed with an echocardiographic criterion (Pearson et al., 2000). The new definition based on the presence of 4 criteria is summarized in Table 1.

Classic criteria (Demakis et al., 1971)
1. The development of heart failure in the last month of pregnancy or within the first 5 months postpartum
2. The absence of an identifiable cause for heart failure
3. The absence of recognizable heart disease prior to the last month of pregnancy
Additional criterion (NHLBI & the Office of Rare Disease of NIH, 1997)
4. Left ventricular systolic dysfunction demonstrated by classic echocardiographic criteria (depressed ejection fraction or shortening fraction)

Table 1. Original definition of peripartum cardiomyopathy

In 1999, Hibbard et al. proposed a more precise echocardiographic criterion that parallels those for detecting idiopathic dilated cardiomyopathy (Hibbard et al., 1999) (Table 2). The new definition has been widely accepted and has improved the diagnosis of both ventricular dysfunction and PPCM. The original definition states that PPCM must develop during the last month of pregnancy or within 5 months after delivery. However, several reports described females who presented with clear PPCM symptoms earlier during pregnancy (Alvarez, 2001; Brown, 1992; Forssell, 1994; Rizeq, 1994; Yahagi, 1994). In 2005, Elkayam et al. provided the largest retrospective database, challenging the classic criteria when they found that clinical course and outcome of females with pregnancy-associated cardiomyopathy diagnosed earlier than the last gestational month are similar to those of females with traditional PPCM. The authors concluded that these two conditions might represent a continuum of a spectrum of the same disease (Elkayam et al., 2005). Since then, several definitions have been proposed (Table 2).

In 2010, the experts considered the modification of the first criterion might be necessary. This definition specifically excludes females who develop cardiomyopathy early in their pregnancy and emphasizes that not all cases of PPCM present with LV dilation. In addition, it is recommended that other conditions which may be exacerbated and associated with heart failure in the puerperium, are excluded before the diagnosis of PPCM is considered. However, in clinical practice, it remains difficult to distinguish females with preexisting asymptomatic cardiomyopathy, progressing during pregnancy and labor, from actual PPCM females (Sliwa et al., 2010a).

Ever since the early descriptions of PPCM, the condition has been defined by several confusing names, such as post-partum heart failure, post-partum myocarditis, Meadow's syndrome, idiopathic myocardial degeneration associated with pregnancy, Zaria syndrome, toxic post-partum heart disease, or recently, postpartal heart disease, post-partum cardiomyopathy or peripartum cardiomyopathy.

Hibbard et al., 1999	NHLBI definition and a strict ecocardiographic criterion of left ventricular (LV) dysfunction: 1. ejection fraction < 45% or fractional shortening < 30% 2. end-diastolic dimension > 2.7cm/m²
American Heart Association [AHA] Scientific Statement on contemporary definitions and classifications of the cardiomyopathies (Maron et al., 2006)	A rare and dilated acquired primary cardiomyopathy associated with LV dysfunction and heart failure
European Society of Cardiology [ESC] on the classification of cardiomyopathies (Dickstein et al., 2008)	A non-familial, non-genetic form of dilated cardiomyopathy associated with pregnancy
Heart Failure Association of the ESC Working Group on PPCM (Sliwa et al., 2010a)	An idiopathic cardiomyopathy presenting with heart failure secondary to LV systolic dysfunction *towards the end of pregnancy or in the months following delivery*, where no other cause of heart failure is found. It is a diagnosis of exclusion. The LV may not be dilated but the ejection fraction is nearly always reduced below 45%

Table 2. Definitions of peripartum cardiomyopathy

Peripartum cardiomyopathy is the preferred term because it highlights the overall chronological spectrum of the disease (Abboud et al., 2007). Another accepted term is *pregnancy-associated cardiomyopathy* or *early peripartum cardiomyopathy*, used for those females with cardiomyopathy developing heart failure before the last month of pregnancy or at least five months after delivery (Ntobeko et al., 2009). These cases may be subclinical dilated cardiomyopathies presenting the first symptoms in early pregnancy, or viral myocarditis, both distinct entities from PPCM (Pyatt & Dubey, 2011).

3. Epidemiology

Good data about incidence are unavailable because so few population-based registries exist. Most studies have been performed in South Africa, Haiti, and USA, but PPCM was also reported in Caucasian, Japanese, Chinese, Indian, and Korean women. Until recently, only small prospective studies reporting the experience of single centers were available to estimate the incidence of the disease (Desai et al., 1995; Fett et al., 2002, 2005a; Pyatt & Dubey, 2011). Only two large retrospective population-based studies have been conducted in USA to identify cases of PPCM. Mielniczuk et al. reported an estimated incidence of 1:3189 live births, with a trend toward an increase over the study period (1 case/2289 live births for the years 2000-2002), probably related to increasing maternal age and rates of multiple births or to increasing recognition and diagnosis of the disease (Mielniczuk et al., 2006). The second study was performed by Brar et al., who reported an incidence of 1:4025 live births (Brar et al., 2007). The estimates are almost similar for Japan and Australia. PPCM is sporadic in Europe in the white women (Bahloul et al., 2009; Ramaraj & Sorell, 2009). The estimated in-hospital mortality due to PPCM in USA is 1.36% in more recent reports, less than in older series, perhaps due in part to high utilization of modern heart failure therapy (Mielniczuk et al., 2006). These more recent data from the United States suggest a significant difference in the incidence between certain ethnic groups. The lowest observed incidence is reported in Hispanics and the highest in African-Americans (Brar et al., 2007). Outside the United States, the most comprehensive data come from the Peripartum Cardiomyopathy Project in Haiti, which estimates the incidence of PPCM as high as 1case/299 live births (Fett et al., 2005a). The data have been confirmed by Gentry et al., who noted an incidence of 1 case/1000 live births in South Africa (Gentry et al, 2010). In fact, in the absence of a multicentric trial, the incidence varies widely between African countries. For example, in Tunisia the reported incidence is very low unlike Nigeria where older studies have reported 1 case/100 live births (Bahloul et al., 2009).

On the basis of several reports series of PPCM, varying genetic pools and diverse environmental factors have been proposed as risk factors in different areas. Although not clearly delineated, there are several suggested risk factors for development and recurrence of PPCM (Bahloul et al., 2009; Demakis et al., 1971; Fett et al., 2005a; Fisher et al., 2008; Murali & Baldisseri, 2005; Moioli et al., 2010; Nkoua et al., 1991; Ntusi & Mayosi, 2009; Pearson et al., 2000; Sliwa 2006a, 2006b):

-    African race – appears to be the strongest risk factor, possibly due to a greater incidence of arterial hypertension in this group. Brar et al. reported the incidence of PPCM in African-American women to be 2.9-fold higher than in whites, and 7-fold than in Hispanics (Brar et al., 2007). Recently, Elkayam has shown that PPCM in USA is not limited to African women (Elkayam et al., 2005). It remains unclear whether race represents an independent risk factor.

-    advanced maternal age – the disease generally occurs over the age of 30 years;

-    multiparity – 71% of cases occur after ≥ 3 pregnancies compared with 8% in primigravidas (Demakis, 1971, as cited in Ntusi, 2009);

-    twin pregnancies – which are observed in 8-13% of cases compared with 1-2% rate noted among healthy women;

-    gestational hypertension – with an incidence of approximately 43%, substantially higher than the 8% to 10% incidence in the overall pregnant population. It is important to note that pregnancy-related hypertensive disorders should be considered as distinct entities from PPCM, and not included in the spectrum of PPCM. The complete recovery of LV function in pregnancy-related hypertensive disorders is the rule, whereas persistent cardiac dysfunction is frequent in PPCM patients.

-    prolonged use of tocolytics refers to the use of terbutaline, salbutamol, ritodrine, isoxsuprine, magnesium sulfate etc for a period of at least four weeks (Bassett, 1985 as cited in Ntusi, 2009). The association with left ventricular dysfunction seems to be unique to pregnancy, as the same drugs do not determine similar complications in non-pregnant patients, even at high doses.

-    certain cultural practices performed during the puerperium which are frequently related with high incidence of PPCM, such as consuming lake salt or rock salt known as "kanwa" (to promote the flow of breast milk), or heating of the body on a clay bed with a fire beneath to keep warm (Moioli et al., 2010; Murali & Baldisseri, 2005);

-    socio-economic level is discussed as a risk factor, and can be summarized in a stereotyped profile: "poor African female, with malnutrition and multiparity, making strenuous and sustained physical effort during pregnancy" (Bahloul et al., 2009).

Main concerns

What is the true incidence? Physicians still do not know how often PPCM occurs. Despite being a rare disease in many geographic areas of the world, PPCM remains an important cause of morbidity and mortality in pregnant females.

Who is at risk? There are several cardiac factors that may play a causative role. Regardless of the documented risk factor, the association with PPCM is not clearly explained.

Implications for research

Collaborative, multicenter, prospective, population-based, well-conducted trials are required for adequate diagnosis of this condition.

---

4. Etiology and pathogenesis

Despite extensive research into its underlying etiology and pathogenesis, it is not clear exactly how PPCM occurs (Ntusi et al., 2009).

Previously, PPCM was generally considered a form of idiopathic dilated cardiomyopathy that was unmasked by the hemodynamic stress of pregnancy (Cunningham et al., 1986). In this case, one would expect PPCM to present during the second trimester coincident with the maximum hemodynamic load of pregnancy. However, it more commonly presents later in pregnancy or postpartum. Moreover, 30% of patients with PPCM experience complete recovery, with partial recovery in many cases, in contrast to rare recovery in idiopathic dilated cardiomyopathy (Fett et al., 2002). Finally, epidemiological data show that PPCM is diagnosed in young women during the peripartum period, whereas idiopathic dilated cardiomyopathy is more common in older patients (Pearson et al., 2000). Although the two conditions have similar clinical presentations and hemodynamic features, there are also significant differences in histological characteristics.

It is now accepted that PPCM is a distinct entity, rather than a clinically silent underlying cardiomyopathy exacerbated by the hemodynamic changes during pregnancy (Robson et al., 1989).

The pathogenetic mechanisms of PPCM have been difficult to study as its incidence is too low to allow meaningful evaluations, and the suitable animal models to study the disease are rare. Several hypotheses have been proposed (Figure 1), but at the present time, two hypotheses are foremost: pregnancy associated hormonal changes, specifically the role of prolactin, and viral infection.

4.1 Excessive prolactin production

Pregnancy is a physiological state associated with enhanced oxidative stress related to high metabolic turnover and elevated tissue oxygen requirements. In order to protect the heart, an efficient antioxidant defense mechanism counteracts the oxidative stress. The total antioxidant capacity increases in the last trimester with a peak early postpartum (Toescu et al., 2002).

Prolactin has been suggested as a potential mechanism in the development of PPCM (Kothari, 1997). Experimental data in a mouse model of PPCM demonstrates the activation of STAT3 pathway by 23-kDa prolactin to be necessary (Hilfiker-Kleiner et al., 2007a). STAT3 is a cardiac tissue-specific DNA-binding protein, activator of transcription-3 that promotes myocardial angiogenesis and cardiomyocyte hypertrophy. In addition,

STAT3 protects the heart from pregnancy-induced oxidative stress in part by up-regulation of a powerful reactive oxygen species, scavenging mitochondrial enzyme named manganese superoxide dismutase (MnSOD) (Negoro et al., 2001). Reduced levels of STAT3 lead to an unbalanced peri/postpartum oxidative stress, a potent stimulus for the activation of prolactin-cleaving protease catehpsin D in cardiomyocytes. The result is cleavage of the nursing hormone prolactin into an antiangiogenic, proapoptotic, and proinflammatory 16-kDa subfragment (Roberg & Ollinger, 1998). Interestingly, prolactin is a hormone with opposing cardiovascular effects, depending on the circulating form. The full-length 23-kDa prolactin had no adverse effects on the heart (Hilfiker-Kleiner et al., 2007a). In contrast, high expression of 16-kDa fragment destroys the cardiac microvasculature, reduces in vivo cardiac function, promotes ventricular dilatation. The same fragment inhibits vascular endothelial growth factor-induced proliferation of endothelial cells and migration, induces apoptosis, dissociation of capillary structures, impairs nitric oxide-mediated vasorelaxation, and cardiomyocyte function (Hilfiker-Kleiner et al., 2008). Prolactin production is not limited to pituitary gland, various other cell types, such as fibroblasts, being able to produce it (Nagafuchi et al., 1999). PPCM is often associated with a high degree of cardiac fibrosis mediated by locally produced prolactin, which enhances the circulating pituitary 16-kDa prolactin damaging cardiac effects.

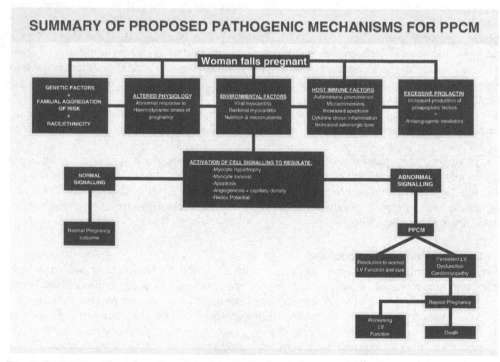

Fig. 1. Summary of proposed pathogenic mechanisms for PPCM (from Ntusi, N.B.A. & Mayosi, B.M. Aetiology and risk factors of peripartum cardiomyopathy: A systematic review. *Int J Cardiol*, Vol.131, No.2 (Jan 2009), pp. 168-179, with permission from Elsevier)

There is more evidence linking findings from experimental models to human PPCM. Patients with acute PPCM have increased serum levels of oxidized low-density lipoprotein indicative for enhanced oxidative stress, activated cathepsin D, and 16-kDa prolactin compared with pregnancy matched healthy controls (Hilfiker-Kleiner et al., 2007a). It is therefore likely that activation of this cascade plays a key functional role in human PPCM. PPCM patients have also significantly elevated pro-apoptotic serum markers (e.g. soluble death receptor sFas/Apo-1) with predictive power of impaired functional status and mortality (Sliwa et al., 2006b). In explanted terminally failing hearts from PPCM patients, low STAT3 protein levels are displayed, suggesting the role of this signaling pathway in the pathogenesis (Hilfiker-Kleiner et al., 2007a) (Figure 2).

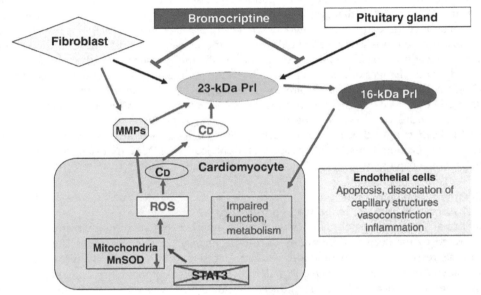

Fig. 2. Schematic mechanism for the development of PPCM (from Hilfiker-Kleiner, D., Sliwa, K. & Drexler, H. (2008). Peripartum Cardiomyopathy: Recent Insights in its Pathophysiology. *Trends Cardiovasc Med,* Vol.18, No.5 (July 2008), pp. 173–179; with permission from Elsevier)

Consistent with the idea of prolactin involvement, blockade by bromocriptine, a dopamine D2 receptor agonist, was tested. Bromocriptine eliminates the substrate for the generation of 16-kDa prolactin, and prevents the onset of disease in the mouse model of PPCM (Hilfiker-Kleiner et al., 2007a) (Figure 2). Several reports suggest that bromocriptine may have beneficial effects when added to the standard therapy of heart failure in women with acute onset of PPCM (Habedank et al., 2008; Hilfiker-Kleiner et al., 2007b; Sliwa et al., 2010b). However, at present, bromocriptine is not recommended until results of ongoing controlled randomized trials will provide information for the actual benefit of this therapy concept in patients with PPCM.

4.2 Viral myocarditis
The relationship between pregnancy and viral myocarditis was established in 1968 in pregnant mice (Farber & Glasgow, 1970). Myocarditis as a cause of PPCM in humans was

first suggested by Gouley et al., who corroborated infection with enlarged hearts with focal areas of fibrosis and necrosis (Gouley et al., 1937). Since then, several investigators have suggested myocarditis as a cause of PPCM (Cenac, 2003 as cited in Ntusi, 2009; Melvin, 1982; O'Connell, 1986). The prevalence of viruses detected in endomyocardial biopsies varies considerably between the different studies, ranging from less than 10% (Rizeq et al., 1994) to 78% (Midei et al., 1990), with a similar incidence in controls, suggesting no specific role for viral infection in the etiology of PPCM. It is worth noting that the molecular pathological study of endomyocardial biopsies within a cohort with PPCM found a high prevalence of viral genomes (parvovirus B19, human cytomegalovirus and herpes virus 6, Epstein-Barr virus) as well as inflammatory changes consistent with myocarditis (30.7%) (Bultmann et al., 2005). Other investigation suggests that viral infection increases the severity of myocardial damage in postpartum mice in comparison with non-pregnant control subjects (Lyden & Huber, 1984, as cited in Ramaraj & Sorrell, 2009). It is possible that the postviral immune response to be directed inappropriately against native cardiac tissue proteins leading to LV systolic dysfunction in the presence of the characteristic hemodynamic changes during pregnancy. Given the imunosuppressed state of pregnancy, it is logical that pregnant women are more susceptible to infection or viral reactivation (Pearson et al., 2000). At the present time, the exact role of viral infection or reactivation is far from conclusive. No convincing data exist that myocarditis is the primary etiology of PPCM. Further studies using newer technologies such as PCR are needed for detecting actively replicating viruses and myocardial viral load in PPCM (Ntusi et al, 2009) and confirming a pathogenic role.

4.3 Other putative hypotheses
4.3.1 Abnormal immune response to pregnancy
Abnormal immune response to pregnancy is another potential mechanism, probably generated by the decreased immunity during pregnancy (Cruz et al., 2010). The abnormal immune response may be produced after previous exposure immunization from prior pregnancy, or previous exposure to paternal major histocompatibility antigens. A local tissue inflammatory response is induced, followed by releasing of cytokines and a nonspecific innocent bystander myotoxicity and myocarditis (Pearson et al., 2000). Circulating auto-antibodies to selected cardiac tissue proteins were reported by several studies in more than 50% of PPCM patients (Sliwa, 2000, 2006a; Sundstrom, 2002, as cited in Cruz, 2010). Auto-antibodies are associated with increased levels of cytokines (tumor necrosis factor-α, interleukin-6, soluble Fas receptors), and are correlated with dilation of LV and systolic dysfunction (Sliwa et al., 2006b). The circulating auto-antibodies are formed against proteins released after delivery (e.g. actin, myosin), when the degeneration of the uterus occurs, and may cross-react with "target-proteins" found in the maternal myocardium (Freedman, 2004; Jahns, R., 2004). It was reported that in all patients with PPCM, irrespective of geographic location, auto-antibodies against cardiac myosin are non-selectively increased immunoglobulins G (class G and subclasses G1, G2, G3) (Warraich et al., 2005). Other studies have reported the phenomenon called chimerism, when fetal cells of hematopoietic origin reside in maternal serum, but remain undetected because of the weak immunogenicity of paternal haploytpe or maternal altered immunity (Ansari, 2002, as cited in Ramaraj & Sorrell, 2009). If fetal cells lodge in maternal myocardium during pregnancy, it is possible to be recognized as non-self while postpartum immune recovery, and an

abnormal immune response is triggered (Pearson et al., 2000). At the present time, it is unclear if all these data contribute directly to myocardial injury in PPCM, or should be considered as a consequence of the disease.

4.3.2 Citokine-mediated inflammation
Citokine-mediated inflammation is a basic pathophysiological mechanism in heart failure. The vasodepressor pro-inflammatory cytokines, like tumor necrosis factor-α, interleukin-6 and 1, interpheron-γ, expressed at high concentrations result in LV systolic dysfunction and remodeling, fetal gene expression, and cardiomyopathy. Increased levels of the same cytokines, and of hs-C-reactive protein have been reported in the serum of patients with PPCM (Fett, 2004; Sliwa, 2006b). It is still unclear if a true causal link between cytokines and PPCM does exist. If cytokines are involved in the pathogenesis of PPCM, these would prove useful targets for immunomodulatory therapy.

4.3.3 Increased myocyte apoptosis
Increased myocyte apoptosis represents an imbalance between cellular elimination and cellular regeneration. Experimental data suggest that terminally differentiated cardiac myocytes undergo apoptosis as the final common pathway in many cardiomyopathies (Narula, 2000; Wencker, 2003). Transgenic mice develop PPCM when cardiac-specific α-subunit of Gq is over-expressed (Hayakawa, 2003, as cited in Hilfiker-Kleiner, 2008). The Gq subunit is discussed to be responsible for coupling several cell surface receptors to intracellular signaling pathways involved in cardiomyocyte hypertrophy and apoptosis.

The inhibition of caspases, the proteases that mediate apoptosis, has been demonstrated to improve LV systolic function and reduce the mortality in pregnant Gαq mice. Recently, the proapoptotic gene Nix or Bnip3 have been demonstrated to play a key role in peripartum cardiac apoptosis and heart failure (Diwan, 2008, as cited in Hilfiker-Kleiner, 2008). Thus, experimental models, as well as indirect evidence in humans (increased plasma levels of key-proteins like Fas and Fas ligand), provides evidence for a role of apoptosis (Sliwa et al., 2006a). On the other side, the role of cardiomyocyte loss as a general key mechanism seems unlikely, since complete recovery of cardiac function has been observed in PPCM patients. Further studies are needed to evaluate the prevalence and exact role of apoptosis in PPCM patients, as well as the therapeutic value to prevent cardiomyopathy decompensation.

4.3.4 Abnormal response to hemodynamic stress
Abnormal response to hemodynamic stressis a hypothesis that suggests the exaggerated decrease in systolic function of LV in the presence of the cardiovascular changes in pregnancy (Ntusi et al., 2009). The normal hemodynamic changes during pregnancy result in a physiological transient and reversible hypertrophy and enlargement of the LV to meet the needs of the fetus and mother (Geva, 1997, as cited in Ntusi, 2009). These changes normally maintain up to 2-3 weeks postpartum and may persist until the 12th week after delivery. In patients with PPCM, LV anatomy may return to normal, but the contractile reserve is persistently decreased when assessed by dobutamine stress echocardiography (Lampert et al., 1997). Until now, there are no convincing data to support this hypothesis.

4.3.5 Genetic susceptibility

Genetic susceptibilitywas first suggested in the 1960s (Pierce at al., 1963). Since that time, several other documented cases with familial clustering of PPCM, as well as familial reports with familial PPCM and idiopathic dilated cardiomyopathy have been published, suggesting the contribution of genetics (Sliwa et al., 2010a). It is not clearly documented whether these cases meet the criterion of absence of an identifiable cause of heart failure, or whether an inherited idiopathic dilated cardiomyopathy becomes symptomatic because of the hemodynamic changes during pregnancy and after delivery. Also, the very high incidence in certain geographic regions or communities is strongly suggestive for environmental factors role. A genetic mutation cannot be excluded, but genetic testing is not usually performed in PPCM. Secondly, experimental studies have reported a genetic susceptibility to viral myocarditis in animals deficient in transforming growth factor-β, as well as the potential role of the defective STATE3 gene, or gene polymorphism of MnSOD (Hilfiker-Kleiner, 2008; Horwitz, 2007; Kim, 2005; Kühl 2005b; Lang 2008). Recently, van Spaendonck-Zwarts et al. investigated the occurrence of PPCM in 90 families with idiopathic dilated cardiomyopathy. The authors suggested that a subset of PPCM could be an initial manifestation of the disease, when a mutation in the gene encoding cardiac troponin C was identified (van Spaendonck-Zwarts et al., 2010). In another study from the USA, Morales et al. confirmed PPCM in 5 cases with gene mutations. The involved genes encoded myosin heavy chain 7 (MYH7), sodium channel, voltage-gated, type V, α-subunit (SCN5A), and presenilin 2 (PSEN2) in 3 cases with familial disease and myosin heavy chain 6 (MYH6), cardiac troponin T2 (TNNT2) in 2 with sporadic disease (Morales et al., 2010). Both reports have important implications, suggesting the necessity for the cardiologic screening in first-degree family members of PPCM patients without recovery of LV function and dimensions. In addition, reproductive risk counseling about PPCM or pregnancy-associated cardiomyopathy is appropriate for first-degree family members of patients with idiopathic dilated cardiomyopathy in the context of a genetic evaluation (Hershberger et al., 2009).

4.3.6 Malnutrition

Malnutrition was thought to be involved because of increased incidence of PPCM in communities with low socio-economic level (Hull, 1937, as cited in Ntusi, 2009; Walsh, 1965). For example, selenium deficiency has been reported in Sahel region of Africa (Cenac et al., 1992) but not in Haiti, and excessive consumption of salt in Nigeria (Ntusi et al., 2009). However, malnutrition it is not a key factor because many cases of PPCM are reported in well-nourished cohorts.

4.3.7 Abnormal hormonal regulation

Abnormal hormonal regulation although proposed in the 1930s, cannot be affirmed (Musser, 1938, as cited in Ntusi, 2009). Estrogens and relaxin were believed to play a role in PPCM, due to the cardiovascular effects, but no convincing evidence has been documented.

4.3.8 Increased adrenergic tone

Increased adrenergic tone secondary to physical or emotional stress has been proposed to cause "myocardial stunning" and transient cardiac dysfunction, fluid overload, decreased colloid osmotic pressure (Wittstein et al., 2005). Considering the evidence for the role of β1-

adrenergic receptor antibodies, it is possible to contribute to cardiac muscle dysfunction (Jahns R., 2004; Freedman, 2004).

4.3.9 Vascular disease
Vascular disease with subsequent myocardial ischemia has also been suggested, but morphology and function of coronary arteries were unaffected in PPCM patients (Koide, 1972; Lampert, 1995, as cited in Cruz, 2010).

4.3.10 Other possible mechanisms
Other possible mechanisms postulate the role of cardiac nitric oxide synthase, cardiac dystrophin, immature dendritic cells, toll-like receptors etc (Ramaraj & Sorell, 2009).

Main concern

What causes PPCM? Contributing factors and specific mechanisms remain unclear. Although various hypotheses have been proposed, so far no cause has been clearly identified. It is likely that PPCM is a heterogenous disorder, with a multifactorial etiology and complex biopathological processes.

Implications for research

Further studies are needed to elucidate this difficult condition. "The challenge will be to devise a study with sufficient power to give valid results" (Fett, 2010).

---

5. Diagnosis

5.1 Clinical presentation
Patients with PPCM present with classical signs and symptoms of systolic heart failure due to other cardiomyopathies. The most common symptoms are dyspnea and fatigue (90%), tachycardia (62%), and peripheral edema (60%) (Elkayam et al., 2005). Other symptoms like persistent nocturnal dry cough, orthopnea, paroxysmal nocturnal dyspnea are frequently reported (Moioli et al., 2010). NYHA class III or IV functional status seem to be the most common initial presentation (Desai et al., 1995). Other non-specific signs and symptoms include dizziness, non-specific praecordial pain (50%), abdominal discomfort, palpitations, most frequently due to tachycardia or supraventricular tachiarryhtmias (Bertrand, 1977; de Beus, 2003; Weinblatt, 1995). Complex ventricular arrhythmias and cardiac arrest have also been reported (Diao et al., 2004). Some case series describe unusual presentations such as acute cyanosis (Cole et al., 2001), multiple thromboembolic events (Carlson et al., 2000) or liver failure (Fussell et al., 2005). Systemic and pulmonary embolic episodes are found during the clinical course of PPCM more frequently than in patients with other forms of cardiomyopathy (Bennani, 2003; Box, 2004; Helms & Kittner, 2005; Jha, 2005; Lasinska-Kowara, 2001). Sudden dyspnea, pleuritic pain, and hemoptysis suggest an episode of pulmonary embolism.

Regarding the physical signs in PPCM, a high incidence of the third heart sound (92%) and displaced apical impulse (72%) are reported (Desai et al., 1996). New murmurs consistent with mitral and tricuspid regurgitation are present in almost 50% of PPCM patients (Fadouach et al., 1994). Sinus tachycardia is the rule of cardiac exam. In the later stages, signs of pulmonary hypertension, including a loud or split second heart sound and pulmonary crackles, are common. Elevated jugular venous pressure and hepatomegaly associated with edema are present as signs of congestive heart failure. Blood pressure may be normal or increased (when gestational hypertension is associated). In the later stages, postural hypotension can occur (Sliwa et al., 2010a). A latent form of PPCM without overt clinical symptoms has been reported (Elkayam et al., 2005).

The clinical diagnosis still represents a challenge because symptoms of early heart failure such as dyspnea, fatigue, palpitations, pedal edema, can appear in normal late pregnancy and after delivery. Therefore, in many cases, patients and their physicians may consider the symptoms to be normal.

There are some important clues for making the diagnosis. Clinical exam remains essential because a persistent sinus tachycardia, third heart sound, basal pulmonary crackles, and elevated jugular venous pressure are abnormal for pregnancy state and heart failure may be considered. Secondly, the diagnosis should be considered whenever women experience unexplained heart failure symptoms and signs during the last month of pregnancy or within 5 months following delivery, in accordance with PPCM definition. It is important to note that 78% of PPCM cases develop heart failure symptoms in the first 4 months after delivery, and only 9% of patients present in the last month of pregnancy (Lampert et al., 1995). It is possible that some patients to present later in postpartum because their symptoms are not initially recognized as heart failure (Sliwa et al., 2010a). Interestingly, Fett et al. reported clinically normal postpartum in Haitian women with asymptomatic echocardiographic systolic dysfunction, who either developed dilated cardiomyopathy or completely recovered LV function (Fett et al., 2005b). These cases may represent a latent phase of PPCM before the development of dilated cardiomyopathy later in life or subclinical dilated cardiomyopathy presenting in early pregnancy or a viral myocarditis, distinct conditions from true PPCM (Fett, 2008; Pyatt &Dubey, 2011). Thirdly, the rapid onset of heart failure symptoms in the peripartum period may also distinguish this clinical entity and requires further investigations.

In conclusion, there are no specific criteria for differentiating symptoms of early heart failure from normal late pregnancy, so it is imperative to maintain a high index of suspicion in conjunction with timing of symptoms to identify the patients with PPCM.

5.2 Investigation of peripartum cardiomyopathy

Blood tests should be done in all patients, although none of these can help in screening or positive diagnosis of PPCM. Initial laboratory assessment should include complete blood count and biochemical parameters. The thyroid function, a septic screen, and viral serology should also be performed in order to exclude other causes of cardiomyopathy and heart failure (Pyatt &Dubey, 2011). Molecular markers of an inflammatory process are found in most of the patients. It was reported that 90% of the patients with PPCM had high levels of plasma C-reactive protein, positively related with LV dimensions and inversely with LV ejection fraction (Fett, 2005a; Sliwa, 2006b). Cardiac markers, such as troponin T determined early after the onset of PPCM, are suggested to have prognostic significance. Only B-type natriuretic peptide (BNP) and N-terminal pro-BNP (NT-proBNP), commonly increased in patients with PPCM, are recommended by the Heart Failure Association of the ESC Working Group on PPCM to be determined (Sliwa et al., 2010a). Measurement of natriuretic peptides can be also helpful for risk stratification and volume status assessment. Increased levels in pregnancy have been related with systolic dysfunction, increased LV filling pressures and LV hypertrophy, acute myocardial infarction (Hameed, 2009; Garrison, 2005).

Genetic testing is not recommended as a routine, but only for research purposes (Sliwa et al., 2010a).

Electrocardiogram is seldom normal in patients with heart failure caused by PPCM, but it is mostly non-specific. Sinus rhythm or sinus tachycardia are usually present, atrial fibrillation or ventricular tachycardia may occur, particularly if LV systolic dysfunction becomes chronic (Diao, 2004; Duran, 2008). An intraventricular block pattern or prolonged PR and QRS are seldom reported. LV hypertrophy pattern, Q waves in the anteroseptal leads, ST-T abnormalities largely vary in incidence between studies (Brown, 1998; O'Connell, 1986, as cited in Moioli, 2010). Negative T waves can be of ischemic origin in 50% of cases (Bertrand, 1975, as cited in Bahloul, 2009).

Chest X-ray should be part of the initial assessment of all patients with PPCM and clinical heart failure. Radiological findings can be cardiomegaly, pulmonary congestion/edema, and pleural effusion.

Echocardiography is the most widely used imaging method, which provides valuable, reproducible diagnostic and prognostic information. The technique is not diagnostic for PPCM, but is important to exclude other causes of heart failure. Hibbard et al. proposed precise echocardiographic criteria that should be applied (**Table 2**). Several studies highlighted the strong relation between LV end-diastolic diameter > 60 mm, or ejection fraction < 30% and the recovery of LV function (Duran, 2008; Elkayam, 2005). Another important finding may be the presence of LV thrombus, particularly when LV function is severely depressed. It is important to note that LV dilatation is not always present (Kane, 2001; Sliwa, 2000). It is strongly recommended to monitor the evolution under treatment before patient's discharge, at 6 weeks, 6 months, and annually (Sliwa et al., 2010a).

Cardiac magnetic resonance imaging (MRI) is widely used in other forms of cardiomyopathy for assessment of cardiac structure and function as a reference technique. Also it has a high ability to detect myocardial fibrosis as a consequence of myocarditis, using delayed contrast enhancement technique with gadolinium. In PPCM, cardiac MRI provides more accurate quantification of chamber volumes and ventricular function, and is more sensitive in detecting LV thrombus than echocardiography (Mouquet, 2008; Srichai, 2006). At the present time, there are four case series with PPCM assessed by cardiac MRI (Caballero-Borrego, 2008; Kawano, 2008; Leurent, 2009; Mouquet, 2008). In only two of these studies the technique revealed myocardial inflammation. Baruteau et al. consider that all these MRI results are not in contradiction, but underline the complex pathogenesis of PPCM. Cardiac MRI can distinguish two forms of PPCM, inflammatory and non-inflammatory, according to the presence or absence of late gadolinium enhancement. Therefore, cardiac MRI can be helpful at initial presentation to conduct further etiologic investigations (Baruteau et al., 2010). The interest for the technique is also suggested by the ability to differentiate PPCM from other forms of cardiomyopathy, like Tako-Tsubo or ischemic cardiomyopathy. The technique might be a useful method for guiding biopsy to the abnormal area (Leurent et al., 2009), and for prognostic stratification (Kawano et al., 2008). In his comment, Fett supports cardiac MRI for PPCM which is not responding to conventional therapy as long as late gadolinium enhancement is more likely to be present in these cases (Fett, 2009). In other words, cardiac MRI could guide the immunosuppressive therapy in the inflammatory forms of PPCM, as this option of treatment has successfully been tested in "myocarditis-like" PPCM (Ntusi et al., 2009). Further larger prospective studies are needed to evaluate these findings, and the real diagnostic contribution of MRI in PPCM. The Heart Failure Association of the ESSC Working Group on PPCM recommends cardiac MRI to be performed at 6 and 12 months for a better assessment of cardiac functional changes (Sliwa et al., 2010a). It remains the problem of using gadolinium during pregnancy, not recommended by the European Society of Radiology until after delivery, unless absolutely necessary (Webb et al., 2005).

Invasive evaluation including cardiac catheterization and coronary angiography are not routinely indicated, as no specific findings are present, and coronary arteries are usually normal in PPCM.

Endomyocardial biopsy is not routinely recommended in PPCM for multiple reasons. Its role is controversial because a specific microscopic pattern for PPCM does not exist, even though a "myocarditis-like" form is frequently found (Fett, 2006a; Zimmermann, 2005). In addition, the technique is not widely available, is invasive, and has a relatively high complication rate.

Considering all these data, PPCM should be suspected whenever the patient experiences symptoms and signs of heart failure during peripartum period. A careful history and physical exam should be performed to identify heart failure due to other cardiac or non-cardiac entities. The differential diagnosis of PPCM should include all the pre-existing clinical conditions, either unrecognized, such as congenital heart disease, or unmasked by pregnancy, such as sporadic and familial idiopathic dilated cardiomyopathies, HIV/AIDS cardiomyopathy, valvular heart disease, particularly rheumatic mitral valve disease. Other non-cardiac conditions (collagen vascular disease, sexually transmitted disease, thyroid disorders) and precipitating factors (current use of alcohol, tobacco, illicit drugs, sodium intake, other therapies) may be also considered. A useful clue for diagnosis is the onset of symptoms, most frequently in postpartum for PPCM unlike the other clinical conditions, which usually present by the 2nd trimester. Pregnancy-associated myocardial infarction, venous thromboembolism, hypertensive heart disease must be also included in the diagnostic approach. Timely diagnosis of PPCM is critical for best outcomes of survival and recovery. Very recently, Fett proposed a screening tool for early diagnosis of PPCM. The test is a focused medical history for PPCM screening, looking for the most common early signs and symptoms of heart failure during last month of pregnancy (Fett, 2011). The author proposes 6 clinical categories, easy to quantify, which are included in a self-scoring system (Table 3). A score ≥ 5 has always been associated with LV systolic dysfunction. A score > 4 suggests the need for further investigation. In this case, a blood BNP test and an echocardiography are recommended. If the score is < 4 the patient should be monitored for BNP and C-reactive protein levels. If increased levels, echocardiography should be performed. The author emphasizes that this test is not diagnostic for PPCM, but encourages an expanded use, because it may be a useful tool for early recognition of the new onset heart failure.

In conclusion, the diagnostic work-up should focus on precise echocardiographic identification of new LV systolic dysfunction, peptide natriuretic measurement (Murali, 2005; Pearson, 2000), and ruling out other causes of heart failure. Additional investigations should be based on clinical suspicion. PPCM remains a *diagnosis of exclusion*. Early detection is critically important to the patient with PPCM, because delayed diagnosis may be associated with increased morbidity and mortality (Fett, 2008; Fussell, 2005; Pearson, 2000; Sliwa, 2006a).

Sign/symptom	Characterstics	Scoring
Orthopnea (difficulty breathing when lying flat)	None	0
	Need to elevate head	1
	Need to elevate $\geq 45^0$	2
Dyspnea (shortness of breath on exertion)	None	0
	Climbing 8 or more steps	1
	Walking on level	2
Unexplained cough	None	0
	At night	1
	Day and night	2
Swelling lower extremities	None	0
	Below knee	1
	Above and below knee	2
Excessive weight gain (during last month of pregnancy)	< 2 pounds/week	0
	2-4 pounds/week	1
	> 4 pounds per week	2
Palpitations (sensation of irregular heart beats)	None	0
	When lying down at night	1
	Day and night, any position	2

Table 3. Self-test for early diagnosis of heart failure in PPCM (adapted from Fett JD, 2011).

Main concerns

How to optimize the diagnosis? Early involvement of a cardiologist is needed for a timely diagnosis. The rapid onset of heart failure symptoms in the peripartum period may distinguish this difficult entity, only if other causes of cardiomyopathy are excluded. A screening clinical self-test for early recognition of PPCM is now proposed. Cardiac MRI is also suggested to have a great diagnostic and prognostic potential.

What's next in PPCM investigation?

A multicentre registry systematically using these tools may be considered for a better diagnostic approach.

6. Management of peripartum cardiomyopathy

When considering treatment during the peripartum period, a multidisciplinary approach is needed. Involvement of a maternal-fetal medical team, including a cardiologist, obstetrician, anesthetist, intensivist, and neonatologist is imperative as earliest as possible after the diagnosis. The type of monitoring and care should be individualized to minimize maternal and fetal morbidity and mortality.

6.1 General management of peripartum cardiomyopathy

The medical treatment is generally similar to that for other forms of non-ischemic dilated cardiomyopathy, with some possible exceptions because of the risks of certain drugs on the fetus and newborn. The aims of medical treatment should be to reduce cardiac afterload and preload, while increasing myocardial contractility, to prevent complications, particularly thromboembolism, cardiac arrhythmia, progressive heart failure, and to improve long-term prognosis. Current therapeutic options consist of conventional supportive treatment for acute and chronic heart failure.

6.1.1 Management of acute heart failure

The principles of treatment in PPCM are no different than those applying to acute heart failure from other etiologies (Dickstein et al., 2008). A careful bedside clinical assessment may be helpful to identify the hemodynamic profile. Acute heart failure is usually manifested by worsening pulmonary congestion to pulmonary edema and hypoxemia, peripheral congestion with large weight gain, or low output status indicated by signs of hypoperfusion. All patients should be hospitalized and closely monitored.

Oxygen therapy should be promptly administered in order to relieve symptoms, while achieving an arterial oxygen saturation of ≥ 95%. Non-invasive ventilation with a positive end-expiratory pressure of 5-7.5 cm H_2O should be used when necessary. Extracorporeal membrane oxygenation to treat severe pulmonary edema shortly after delivery has been reported to be useful (Yang et al., 2007).

Patients with significant volume overload but adequate perfusion are treated with *intravenous diuretics*, with an initial bolus of furosemide 20-40 mg i.v. Particular potential adverse effects of diuretics were reported during pregnancy, such as pancreatitis, decreased carbohydrate tolerance (Lindheimer & Katz, 1973) bleeding, and hyponatremia in newborns (Ferrero et al., 2003).

Intravenous nitrates may be added when diuretics are inadequate in controlling symptoms. Nitroglycerin starting at 10-20 up to 200 µg/min is safe when systolic blood pressure is > 110 mmHg. Nitroprusside may be used in certain cases, but theoretically, accumulation of its catabolites thiocyanate and cyanide may be harmful to the fetus (Egan et al., 2009). Nesiritide is insufficiently studied in human pregnancy (Cruz et al., 2010).

Inotropic agents can be used without unnecessary delay in patients with low output status or those with persistent congestion despite diuretic and/or vasodilatator therapy. Dobutamine or levosimendan are strongly recommended when needed. Small studies with levosimendan suggest persistent hemodynamic improvement attributable to production of an active long half-life metabolite (OR-1896), and no safety concern, but breast-feeding should be avoided (Benezet-Mazuecos & de la Hera, 2008; De Luca, 2006).

Mechanical ventricular support and cardiac transplantation are needed in patients dependent on inotropic agents, or intra-aortic balloon pump counterpulsation, despite optimal medical strategy. Surgical support with ventricular assist devices may be considered in appropriately selected patients as a bridge to recovery or to cardiac transplantation. Heart Failure Association of the ESC Working Group on PPCM recommends an individualized discussion between experts in such cases, as the optimal strategy in PPCM is not known (Sliwa et al., 2010a). If the type of ventricular assist devices is discussed, two prosthetic ventricles - BiVADs and CardioWest TAH, depending on body surface area, heart size and presence of multiorgan failure were proposed (Zimmerman et al., 2010). Complications may occur with ventricular assist devices, such as a high incidence of thrombotic events (Potapov et al., 2008). Recovery of myocardial function can occur in approximately 15% of patients with PPCM on ventricular assist device support (Murali et al., 2005). If the clinical improvement does not occur, cardiac transplantation should be considered. Since 1987, when Aravot et al. reported their first experience (Aravot, 1987, as cited in Abboud, 2007), several case series were treated by heart transplantation with mixed results. In 1994, Keogh et al. demonstrated no difference in survival rates for cardiac transplantation in women with dilated cardiomyopathy, irrespective of etiology, but higher rates of early rejection in PPCM were noted (Keogh, 1994, as cited in Zimmerman, 2010). Other authors supported the hypothesis of an overactive immunological response in "myocarditis-like" PPCM, which predisposes to recurrent severe rejection, and subsequent development of fatal transplant-associated complications. A recent prospective study demonstrated that survival and freedom from cardiac allograft vasculopathy in PPCM was similar to that of women with other indications for heart transplantation (Rasmusson et al., 2007). At the present time, based on available data, 0-11% PPCM patients undergo heart transplantation, with a similar outcome compared with other etiologies of heart failure (Sliwa et al., 2010a). Generally, heart transplantation in PPCM is associated with survival rates similar to that in patients with idiopathic dilated cardiomyopathy (88% at 2 years, and 78% at 5 years) (Murali et al., 2005).Very recently, a long term survey on 8 patients with PPCM (mean post-transplant survival 7.1 years) has shown that cardiac transplantation alone can be a successful option (Zimmerman et al., 2010).

6.1.2 Management of stable heart failure

There are no clinical trials to support any particular treatment regimen for PPCM. After delivery, the patient should be treated according to the current guidelines for heart failure (Pearson, 2000; Sliwa, 2010a). During pregnancy and lactation, the management approach must consider the welfare of the fetus along with that of the mother, so several restrictions to these guidelines will be applied.

Dietary restrictions and lifestyle changes are essential and complementary to pharmacological therapy. Fluid restriction to ≤ 2 liters per day and salt restriction (2-4 g per day) are advisable for volume overload control, particularly when NYHA class III and IV symptoms occur. Daily monitoring for edema and weight loss is clinically useful (Oakley et al., 2003). Smoking and alcohol cessation is strongly recommended. Strict bed rest was the standard in the past, still not recommended, except the patients with severe symptoms. Regular modest exercise may be resumed after relief of symptoms (Pyatt &Dubey, 2011; Sliwa 2006a). Since many of pharmacological agents are secreted in the breast milk, breast-feeding is not advised in patients with PPCM (Sliwa et al., 2010a).

Diuretics should be used cautiously because of decreasing placental perfusion with aggressive administration (Egan, 2007; Sliwa 2006a). After delivery, diuretics are safe to reduce preload, and relieve symptoms of pulmonary congestion and volume overload (Amos, 2006; Oakley, 2003). Loop diuretics, such as furosemide, are most frequently used and safer during hospitalization. Thiazide diuretics may be added, if loop diuretics are insufficient, or used in mild cases (Oakley, 2003; Sliwa 2010a). Possible increase of risk of births defects or fetal thrombocytopenia, were reported (Cruz et al., 2010). On experimental studies, spironolactone is reported to have antiandrogenic effects during late pregnancy, but it can be safely added in postpartum period (Pyatt &Dubey, 2011). Eplerenone should be also avoided during pregnancy, as its effects on human fetus are insufficiently studied (Muldowney et al., 2009).

Angiotensin-converting enzyme inhibitors (ACEI) and *angiotensin-II receptor blockers* (ARB) are contraindicated, because of severe fetal toxicity in the 2nd and 3nd trimester of pregnancy, particularly on kidney, resulting in oligohydramnios, fetal renal failure, and neonatal death, but also hypocalvaria, limb contractions, hypoplastic lungs (Cruz et al., 2010). After delivery, or in postpartum onset PPCM, ACEI and ARB are efficient agents to reduce the afterload, and are strongly recommended, as it has been demonstrated to improve survival in all patients with systolic heart failure. It is also recommended the patient counseling about the teratogenic potential of these drugs, with a recurrent pregnancy (Cruz et al., 2010). Some of ACEI, such as captopril and enalapril, are safe during breast-feeding (Ghuman et al., 2009).

Hydralazine and long-acting nitrates are considered safe and useful to reduce preload. The combination can replace ACEI/ARB during pregnancy, or if there is drug intolerance, and may be added to standard therapy in symptomatic patients (Moioli et al., 2010). The agents are reported to be especially effective and further increase survival among African-American patients with NYAH II and III class heart failure (Hunt et al., 2009). The combination is also compatible with breast-feeding.

β-blockers have not been tested in PPCM, but have been safely used in pregnancy-induced hypertension. *β1-selective blockers* are preferred, as *β2*-blockade is theoretically reported to have anti-tocolytic effect (Ghuman et al., 2009). The benefit of these drugs to maternal survival usually outweighs the potential risk to the fetus and newborn. The risks consist of growth retardation, resulting in low-birth-weight newborns, hypoglicemia and bradycardia. Therefore, care should be given when these drugs are used in late pregnancy. β-blockers are recommended for all patients with PPCM, unless contraindicated, as these drugs improve symptoms, ejection fraction, and long term prognosis, reduce the risk of arrhythmia and sudden death. Because transient worsening of heart failure may appear with initiation of therapy, patients should be stable, with minimal evidence of volume overload, and doses should be titrated cautiously. Although carvedilol has been shown to improve overall survival in dilated cardiomyopathy, no safety information related to its use during pregnancy are available. Therefore, use of metoprolol is preferred under careful monitoring, as the drug is also compatible with breast-feeding (Abboud, 2007; Cruz, 2010).

Antiarrhythmic drugs, although well tolerated, should be used only in the acute setting, because their safety for fetus cannot be guaranteed. β-blockers are often adequate for treating supraventricular arrhythmias, also in chronic use. Sotalol or amiodarone may be needed, but, considering their systemic side effects during chronic use, are not recommended. Calcium channel blockers, because of their negative inotrop effects, are also not recommended. Ventricular arrhythmias may be frequently life-threatening, and should be managed aggressively. Class I and class II antiarrhythmic agents are not recommended, because the drugs are poorly tolerated and have proarrhythmic effect. Digoxin is safe during pregnancy, even if it crosses the placental barrier. Careful monitoring of serum levels is recommended, because of the narrow therapeutic-to-toxic window. A digoxinemia of ≤ 1-1.2 ng/dl and early use of the drug in symptomatic women with ACEI/ARB contraindications are recommended (Cruz et al., 2010). Digoxin is also secreted in breast milk, but no adverse effect has been described in newborns (Moioli et al., 2010). In appropriate patients, electrical cardioversion may be necessary, after transesophageal echocardiography rules out the presence of a left atrial thrombus.

Antithrombotic therapy is recommended as pregnancy and puerperium are prothrombotic states. In addition, LV dysfunction (particularly ejection fraction < 35%), severely dilated cavities, and mural thrombus, history of venous thromboembolism and atrial fibrillation are associated with an increased risk of thromboembolic events. A recent study of 182 women with PPCM demonstrated an incidence of 2.2% for thromboembolic complications (Goland et al., 2009). VKA antagonists are contraindicated prior to delivery, because of their risk of fetal and neonatal cerebral hemorrhage, and central nervous system anomalies for warfarin. Heparins are considered necessary and preferred, as they do not cross the placental barrier, and are found in breast milk in significant amount. Low-weight molecular heparins are preferred, as they have a lower risk of premature maternal osteoporosis and thrombocytopenia. Also, low-weight heparins have a short half-life, so they can be discontinued at least 12 hours prior to delivery, to prevent maternal hemorrhage, and resumed 12-24 hours after delivery. Currently, low-weight heparins are safely used in weight-adjusted doses. A strictly adaptation using anti-Xa monitoring is necessary in women at extremes of body weight, or with renal disease. Fondaparinux cannot be used during pregnancy, as there are no consistent data. In 5-7 days postpartum, heparin can be replaced with VKA antagonists, even to breast-feeding mothers (Torbicki et al., 2008).

Cardiac resynchronization therapy and implantable cardioverter/defibrillators have individualized indication, otherwise very difficult to decide in the context of the natural history of PPCM and lack of specific data. The main concern is the usefulness of such methods in patients who may not need them, if ventricular function will recover. For this reason, the indication is advisable when LV ejection fraction < 35% persists after 6 months following presentation. Patients with recurrent symptomatic ventricular arrhythmias may be candidates for an implantable defibrillator. If NYHA III and IV heart failure symptoms and a QRS duration > 120 ms are present, cardiac resynchronization may be required (Sliwa et al., 2010a).

Novel therapies are emerging, but the available data are inconsistent and limited.

Immune modulatory therapy in PPCM is not clear, although an immune pathogenesis has been postulated. The beneficial effects of intravenous immunoglobulin therapy have been inconsistently demonstrated by several studies. Likewise, immunosuppressive drugs, such as azathioprine, cyclosporine or steroids, have shown mixed results. For all these reasons, a multicenter prospective clinical trial in PPCM is needed to support use of such agents. Some studies suggested that immunosuppressive drugs might be helpful in patients with active biopsy proven lymphocytic myocarditis, only after active viral infection is excluded (Sliwa, 2006a; Zimmerman, 2005). Also, recent studies demonstrate the role of cardiotrophic viruses in some cases of idiopathic dilated cardiomyopathy (Kühl, 2005a, 2005b), but only one study had demonstrated viral genomic material in endomyocardial biopsy from patients with PPCM (Bultmann et al., 2005). At the present time, the role of immunosuppressive therapy in women with negative biopsies remains unknown. It is important to note that current therapies with ACEI, ARB (Godsel et al., 2003), and β blockers (Pauschinger et al., 2005) may have an additional effect on controlling the overactive immune system in PPCM. Also, immunomodulatory therapy acting on inflammatory cytokine TNF-α may be beneficial. Pentoxifyline, a xanthine agent known to inhibit the production of TNF-α and to prevent apoptosis, has been studied in PPCM. In a prospective study of 59 women with PPCM, 30 treated with pentoxifyline 400 mg three times a day in addition to standard therapy of heart failure, a significant improvement of LV function > 10%, and end-diastolic dimensions, a reduction of mortality rate, and greater increase in functional status, compared with the control group were found (Sliwa et al., 2002).

Bromocriptine therapy

Considering the observations that strongly suggest prolactin cleavage as a specific mechanism for the development of PPCM, specific inhibition of its secretion with bromocriptine, a dopamine D2 receptor agonist, is promising. Thus, bromocriptine might represent a novel specific therapeutic approach to either prevent or treat patients with acute PPCM (Hilfiker-Kleiner et al., 2008). Several case reports demonstrated recovery of LV function after treatment with bromocriptine (Elkayam & Goland, 2010; Habedank, 2008; Hilfiker-Kleiner, 2007b; Jahns, B.G., 2008; Meyer, 2010). Very recently, Sliwa et al. reported the results of a prospective, single-center, randomized, proof-of-concept pilot study of women with newly diagnosed PPCM receiving standard therapy with or without bromocriptine for 8 weeks. The addition of bromocriptine appeared to significantly improve LV function (27% at baseline, to 58% at 6 months, p=0.012), and a composite clinical outcome (Sliwa et al., 2010b). Analyzing these data together, Fett remarked that important details of studies design must be corrected for appropriate results. The author proposes some essential conditions to conduct further trials. Patients included in such trials may be best to have serum cathepsin-D activation, positive test for serum 16-kDa prolactin, and very important, to accept lactation suppression while assuring alternative newborn nutrition (Fett, 2010). Also, Fett suggests that bromocriptine treatment should be limited to those patients with LV ejection fraction < 35%, because of poor prognosis with standard therapy in this category. Concerning the safety of bromocriptine in early postpartum women, there are several reports of myocardial infarction (Hopp et al., 1996), while adding adequate anticoagulant therapy, thromboembolism is not reported in such patients (Meyer, 2010; Sliwa, 2010b). Secondly, there are many reports on myocardial infarction in early postpartum independent from bromocriptine administration (Hilfiker-Kleiner et al., 2008).

The results of these studies may represent breakthroughs in the understanding of PPCM pathogenesis, and in the development of a new specific therapy for this clinical entity. But, at the present time, a large, prospective, multicenter, randomized trial is needed to allow bromocriptine extensive use. Such a trial is on-going in Haiti and South Africa (Pyatt & Dubey, 2011).

Other proposed therapies are based on the potential of several agents, such as calcium channel antagonists, statins, interferon-β, monoclonal antibodies, or methods (immunoadsorbtion, apheresis) to influence pro-inflammatory cytokines in acute myocarditis (Ramaraj & Sorrell, 2009).

Main concern

How to treat better? The current medical strategies are not always safe enough for maternal prognostic. There is no clear evidence for the beneficial effect of standard therapy on the recovery of cardiac function in patients with PPCM. As the cause of PPCM is still unknown, no specific therapy has been established to treat this condition.

Implications for research

As the excessive prolactin hypothesis seems to be specific for PPCM, a specific therapeutic intervention using bromocriptine should be tested in an extensive, controlled manner.

6.2 Specific management of peripartum cardiomyopathy

In addition to treatment of heart failure, an obstetrical plan for close monitoring must be developed when PPCM is diagnosed during pregnancy. A collaborative approach, including the obstetrician, cardiologist, anesthesiologist, and neonatologist is essential to optimal care. Serial clinical assessment should be scheduled during late pregnancy. Antenatal testing, such as non-stress test and amniotic fluid index, or biophysical profile is also recommended (Cruz et al., 2010). A baseline ultrasound scan is best to be performed during pregnancy for monitoring the fetus (Sliwa et al, 2010a). If patient is stable, responsive to medical therapy, the pregnancy should be allowed to go to term. The medical team should discuss the delivery mode, primarily considering the mother's benefit. Spontaneous vaginal delivery is preferred in stable women with healthy fetus. For patients with newly diagnosed PPCM before delivery, labor should be induced, or a cesarean section must be planned if mothers are critically ill, or LV function is deteriorating rapidly, or with obstetrical indication (Murali, 2005). After delivery, strict maintenance of fluid status is recommended, using diuretic therapy to prevent volume overload, as fluids are resorbed into the intravascular space (Cruz et al., 2010). Continuous invasive maternal monitoring, including an arterial line and pulmonary catheter, for adequate assessment of patient's hemodynamic status and guide management, as well as continuous fetal cardiotocography are strongly recommended (de Beus et al., 2003). Antenatal medication may be administered, except heparin which should be discontinued at least 12 hours prior to delivery, and resumed 12-24 hours after delivery, with obstetrician and anesthesiologist's permission. Continuous analgesia and anesthesia are needed to minimize further cardiac stress and pain relief, and should be performed with careful specialized monitoring. Epidural analgesia is preferred during labor, as it stabilizes cardiac output through a sympathectomy-induced afterload reduction (Sliwa et al., 2010a). Continuous spinal anesthesia, with epidural analgesia are recommended for cesarean section, as the hemodynamic stability may be more easily maintained (Murali et al., 2005). If general anesthesia is required, drugs with myocardial depressant effect should be avoided, and induction and maintenance with a high-dose opioid technique is preferred. The second stage of labor can cause maximum hemodynamic and oxidative cardiac stress, so these periods must be shortened using a vacuum device or low forceps. A single dose of intramuscular oxytocin can optimally manage the third stage of labor; ergometrine is forbidden (Oakley et al., 2003).Breastfeeding should be avoided in patients with PPCM, although several drugs have been tested and are safe.

7. Prognosis

7.1 Predictive factors and follow–up

Very few studies have been done to assess the long-term survival and recovery outcomes in PPCM. Although PPCM is a form of dilated cardiomyopathy, a characteristic feature is that a higher rate of spontaneous recovery of LV function occurs. A subset of women with PPCM, despite using an optimal medical treatment, follows a rapid and irreversible course, associated with persistent LV dysfunction, severe heart failure, or premature death.

Whitehead et al. reported that in USA 30-50% of patients return to normal within 6 months post partum (Whitehead et al., 2003), while a single centre prospective study, conducted in South Africa, described only a 23% recovering rate of LV function, despite optimal therapy with ACEI and β blockers (Sliwa et al., 2006b). The same author reported a 32% 6-month mortality rate in case series from South Africa (Sliwa et al., 2000). In another study, in Haitian women, with a mean follow-up period of 5 years, the rate of recovery was 31.5%, while mortality rate was 15 %. An important finding of this study was that the recovery to normal LV function can occur later, after 2-3 years after diagnosis, so it is not limited to the first 6-12 months (Fett et al., 2005a). A recent study describes similar rates of LV function recovery and survival in women from USA, Haiti, and South Africa, probably related to improvements in medical therapy, and to the aggressive use of cardioverters in the non-American studied population (Modi et al., 2009). Analyzing *the predictive factors* for long-term prognostic, Duran et al. concluded NYHA functional class, QRS duration, and LV parameters at the time of diagnosis were important predictors. Initial cut-off values of ≤ 5.5 cm for LV end-systolic diameter, and > 27% for LV ejection fraction were identified to predict complete recovery of LV function, while QRS duration on electrocardiogram ≥ 120 ms was a predictor for mortality (Duran et al., 2008). Reviewing 182 patients with PPCM for major adverse events and death, Goland et al. also demonstrated that in all cases there was a strong relation with severe LV dysfunction, non-Caucasian race, and a delayed diagnosis (Goland et al., 2009). These findings complete previous observations about the relation between the severity and persistence of LV dysfunction and the incidence of morbidity and mortality. A LV ejection fraction > 30% at the time of diagnosis might be a predictor for recovery (Elkayam et al., 2005). LV end-diastolic diameter ≥ 6 cm and fractional shortening ≤ 20% are proposed as risks factors for long-term prognosis, as are correlated with a more than threefold higher risk of progressing to persistent LV dysfunction later on (Chapa, 2005; Wittin, 1997). Recently, Baruteau et al. discussed the potential significance of cardiac MRI in prognostic stratification, by assessing LV size, function, and contractile reserve, as well as prognostic MRI factors identified in myocarditis for "myocarditis-like" forms of PPCM (end-diastolic volume, septal localization, and total amount of late gadolinium enhancement at initial time) (Baruteau et al., 2010). Other authors propose immunological mediators and markers of apoptosis to predict outcome. Elevated C-reactive protein and Fas/APO-1 were reported to be related to decreased LV function and mortality (Sliwa et al., 2006b). These perspectives remain to be evaluated by further studies.

In summary, the prognosis varies according to geographical region, and probably, the most important predictor remains the recovery of LV systolic function.

Follow-up of patients with PPCM is similar with that for other forms of cardiomyopathy and LV systolic dysfunction. Patients should be monitored regularly to assess clinical course, complications, LV systolic dysfunction and dimensions, and the response to treatment. Considering that the recovery interval is not restricted to the first 6-12 months postpartum, it is strongly recommended to continue treatment and follow-up for a long period of time to achieve best results (Fett, 2009). However, the optimal period remains unknown. At the present time, echocardiography is the most important tool for serial assessment. In the first several weeks after diagnosis, an echocardiogram should be performed to assess the level of LV function. After that, it should be repeated at about every 6-12 months until recovery is confirmed, or a plateau is reached (Sliwa et al., 2006a). Dobutamine stress echocardiography may be performed to assess the potential for LV function recovery, by measuring the inotropic contractile reserve (Dorbala et al., 2005). The technique is useful especially when LV systolic function is normal, and the contractile reserve remains decreased (Lampert et al., 1997).

7.2 Subsequent pregnancies, risk of relapse

One of the most important issues in PPCM is the safety of subsequent pregnancies. Even after the full recovery of LV function, the risk of relapse might be present.

In Haitian women, Fett et al. described a rate of recurrence of 53% with subsequent pregnancy. In a retrospective study in USA, it was observed that subsequent pregnancy was associated with the recurrence of heart failure, regardless the previous LV function. However, in women who had a normal LV function, the rate of heart failure was 21% compared with 44% in women who had altered function. Also, all deaths occurred in the last group. Furthermore, recovery of LV function was more frequent in patient with an ejection fraction > 30% at diagnosis of disease (Elkayam et al., 2001). Another retrospective study confirmed a better prognosis for subsequent pregnancy in women who had a higher ejection fraction at diagnosis. However, no relation between ejection fraction and worsening clinical symptoms was found in 29% of patients. Also, a baseline ejection fraction of ≤ 25% at index pregnancy was associated with a higher rate of cardiac transplant (Habli et al., 2008). According to these data, it is especially important to provide the most appropriate information about a potential relapse with subsequent pregnancy. LV systolic function seems to be the key prognostic factor when counseling women with PPCM about the further risks. Individual planning might be done after an echocardiogram was performed:

-   if LV ejection fraction is < 25% at diagnosis or incompletely recovered, the advice should be against further pregnancy (Sliwa et al., 2010a);
-   even if LV function is normal, the patients ought to have stress-echocardiography:
    -   women with an abnormal LV inotropic response to dobutamine have a moderate risk of relapse and pregnancy is not recommended;
    -   women with complete recovery on both echocardiography and dobutamine stress test can be informed about the low rate of complications. In this group, despite a 35% rate of risk of recurrence, pregnancy can be completed in almost all cases (Pyatt & Durbey, 2011).

In postpartum period, it is imperative to give contraceptive counseling and educate the patients about the existent alternatives. Women who had PPCM should avoid pregnancy, best until LV function has recovered. The combined oral contraceptives, containing estrogens and progestins are contraindicated, as estrogens increase the thromboembolic risk. Progesterone contraception alone is permitted (Thorne et al., 2006). Barrier methods are not recommended as they have a high rate of failure. Intrauterine systems are the most efficient and safe methods of contraception. Sterilization methods, including vasectomy, tubal ligation, and insertion of intratubal stents may be considered (Sliwa et al., 2010a).

At the present time, no protocols for decision-making when counseling women with PPCM about risks of subsequent pregnancies are established. For this reason, it is advisable that every women who experienced PPCM, to be considered at risk, and to be closely monitored by the medical team, in a high-risk obstetrical center.

Main concern

What is the course and prognosis of the disease? With the sparse knowledge in this field, the individual outcome is difficult to predict.

Implications for research

Novel diagnostic strategies, based on improved understanding of pathophysiology and molecular basis of PPCM, should be developed to enhance both diagnostic and prognostic utility. Collecting data from the children born to affected women should be an important priority.

---

8. Conclusions and future directions

Since its original description, peripartum cardiomyopathy remains a challenge for both diagnosis and treatment. Although several advances have been made to further the knowledge, the condition is still considered a cardiomyopathy of unknown cause. In terms of future research, a better understanding of its molecular basis and fundamental underlying mechanisms, including potential genetic contribution and life-style aspects, is needed. From a clinical perspective, the ability to identify patients at risk to develop the disease is mandatory. Despite current definition, PPCM can remain undiagnosed until it's too late, as some important issues, such as, its rarity in developed countries, the heterogenity of studied populations, and the lack of adherence to diagnostic guidelines, are not resolved. Collaborative, multicentre prospective, well-conducted, population-based trials are required for the development of national and international health policies on prevention, early diagnosis and management, and standard therapeutic control. The Peripartum Cardiomyopathy Netwotk is a NIH-funded North America ongoing trial conducted in order to address some of unresolved issues, as long as the Haitian PPCM Registry is the only existing population-based registry in the world (Fett, 2005a, 2010). Novel diagnostic strategies and biomarkers are potential candidates that should be validated in large clinical trials. Cardiac MRI and prolactin production might provide valuable diagnostic and prognostic information. Also, it would be ideal to have some specific therapeutic strategies. The most realistic candidate seems to be bromocriptine, although potential new treatments, including immune-modulatory therapy, apheresis, and antiviral agents might have a decisive role. Considering all these data, it is important for clinicians to be aware of this condition, so that unnecessary delays in diagnosis can be avoided, and appropriate therapy can be prescribed in a timely fashion. With current technology, clinicians and researchers are now connected, and new bases for multidisciplinary collaboration might be developed.

9. References

Abboud, J., Murad, Y., Chen-Scarabelli, C., Saravolatz, L., & Scarabelli, T.M. (2007). Peripartum cardiomyopathy: A comprehensive review. *Int J Cardiol*, Vol.118, No.3, (Jun 2007), pp. 295-303, ISSN 0167-5273

Alvarez Navascues, R., Marin, R., Testa, A., Pañeda, F., & Alvarez-Grande, J. (2001). Preeclampsia and peripartum cardiomyopathy: infrequent association. *Nefrologia*, Vol.21, No.1, (Jan-Feb 2001), pp. 84-87, ISSN 0211-6995

Amos, A.M., Jaber, W.A. & Russell, S.D. (2006). Improved outcomes in peripartum cardiomyopathy with contemporary. *Am Heart J*, Vol.152, No.3 (Sep 2006), pp. 509-513, ISSN 0002-8703

Bahloul, M., Ben Ahmed, M.N., Laaroussi, L., Chtara, K., Kallel H., Dammak, H., Ksibi, H., Samet, M., Chelly, H., Hamida, C.B., Chaari, A., Amouri, H., Rekik, N. & Bouaziz, M. (2009). Myocardiopathie du péripartum: incidence, physiopathologie, manifestations cliniques, prise en charge thérapeutique et prognostic. *Annales Françaises d'Anesthésie et de Réanimation*, Vol.28, No.1 (Jan 2009), pp 44-60, ISSN 0750-7658

Baruteau, A.E., Leurent, G., Martins, R.P., Thebault, C., Treguer, F., Leclercq, C., Daubert, J.C. & Mabo, P. (2010). Peripartum cardiomyopathy in the era of cardiac magnetic resonance imaging: First results and perspectives. *Int J Cardiol*, Vol.144, No.1, (Sep 2010), pp 143-145, ISSN 0167-5273

Benezet-Mazuecos, J. & de la Hera, J. (2008). Peripartum cardiomyopathy: A new successful setting for levosimendan. *Int J Cardiol*, Vol.123, No.3 (Jan 2008), pp. 346-347, ISSN 0167-5273

Bennani, S.L., Loubaris, M., Lahlou, I., Haddour, N., Badidi, M., Bouhouch, R., Cherti, M. & Arharbi, M. (2003) Postpartum cardiomyopathy revealed by acute lower limb ischemia. *Ann Cardiol Angeiol (Paris)*, Vol.52, No.6 (Dec 2003), pp. 382–385, ISSN 0003-3928

Bertrand, E., Langlois, J., Renambot, J., Chauvet, L. & Ekra, A. (1977). La myocardiopathie du post-partum : à propos de 25 cas. *Arch Mal Coeur Vaiss*, Vol.70, No.2 (Feb 1977), pp 169–178, ISSN 0003-9683

Box, L.C., Hanak, V. & Arciniegas, J.G. (2004). Dual coronary emboli in peripartum cardiomyopathy. *Tex Heart Inst J*, Vol.31, No.4 (Oct-Dec 2004), pp. 442-444, ISSN 0730-2347

Brar, S.S., Khan, S.S., Sandhu, G.K., Jorgensen, M.B., Parkih, N., Hsu, J.W.Y & Shen, A.Y.J. (2007). Incidence, mortality, and racial differences in peripartum cardiomyopathy. *Am J Cardiol*, Vol.100, No.2 (Jul 2007), pp. 302-304, ISSN 0002-9149

Brown, G., O'Leary, M., Douglas, I. & Herkes, R. (1992). Perioperative management of a case of severe peripartum cardiomyopathy. *Anaesth Intensive Care*, Vol.20, No.1 (Feb 1992), pp. 80-83, ISSN 0310-057X

Bultmann, B.D., Klingel, K., Nabauer, M., Wallwiener, D. & Kandolf, R. (2005). High prevalence of viral genomes and inflammation in peripartum cardiomyopathy. *Am J Obstet Gynecol*, Vol.193, No.2 (Aug 2005), pp. 363-365, ISSN 0002-9378

Caballero-Borrego, J., Garcia-Pinilla, J.M., Rueda-Calle, E. & de Teresa-Galvan, E. (2008). Evidence of gadolinium late-enhancement on cardiac magnetic resonance imaging in a patient with peripartum cardiomyopathy. *Rev Esp Cardiol*, Vol.61, No.2 (Feb 2008), pp. 215-222, ISSN 0300-8932

Carlson, K.M., Browning, J.E., Eggleston, M.K. & Gherman, R.R. (2000). "Peripartum cardiomyopathy presenting as lower extremity arterial thromboembolism. A case report," *Journal of Reproductive Medicine for the Obstetrician and Gynecologist*, Vol.45, No.4 (Apr 2000), pp. 351–353, ISSN 0024-7758

Cenac, A., Simonoff, M., Moretto, P. & Djibo, A. (1992). A low plasma selenium is a risk factor for peripartum cardiomyopathy. A comparative study in Sahelian Africa. *Int J Cardiol*, Vol.36, No. (Jul 1992), pp. 57-59, ISSN 0167-5273

Chapa, J.B., Heiburger, H.B., Weinert, L., Decara, J., Lang, R.M. & Hibbard, J.U. (2005). Prognostic value of echocardiography in peripartum cardiomyopathy. *Obstet Gynecol*, Vol.105, No.6 (Jun 2005), pp. 1303–1308, ISSN 0961-2033

Cole, W.C., Mehta, J.B., Roy, T.M. & Downs, C.J. (2001). "Peripartum cardiomyopathy: echocardiogram to predict prognosis," *Tennessee Medicine*, Vol.94, No.4 (Apr 2001), pp. 135–138, ISSN 1088-6222

Cruz, M.O., Briller, J. & Hibbard, J.U. (2010). Update on Peripartum Cardiomyopathy. *Obstet Gynecol Clin N Am*, Vol.37, No.2 (Jun 2010), pp. 283-303, ISSN 0889-8545

Cunningham, F.G., Pritchard, J.A., Hankins, G.D., Anderson, P.L., Lucas, M.J. & Armstrong, K.F. (1986). Peripartum heart failure: idiopathic cardiomyopathy or compounding cardiovascular events? *Obstet Gynecol*, Vol.67, No.2 (Feb 1986), pp. 157-168, ISSN 0300-8835

de Beus, E., van Mook, W.N., Ramsay, G., Stappers, J.L. & van der Putten, H.W. (2003). Peripartum cardiomyopathy: a condition intensivists should be aware of. *Int Care Med*, Vol.29, No.2 (Feb 2003), pp. 167-174, ISSN 0342-4642

De Luca, L., Colucci, W.S., Nieminen, M.S., Massie, B.M. & Gheorghiade, M. (2006). Evidence-based use of levosimendan in different clinical settings. *Eur Heart J*, Vol.27, No.16 (Aug 2006), pp.1908–1920, ISSN 0195-668x

Demakis, J.G., Rahimtoola, S.H., Sutton, G.C., Meadows, W.R., Szanto, P.B., Tobin, J.R. & Gunnar, R.M. (1971). Natural course of peripartum cardiomyopathy. *Circulation*, Vol.44, No.5 (May 1971), pp. 1053-1061, ISSN 0025-619

Desai, D., Moodley, J. & Naidoo, D. (1995). Peripartum cardiomyopathy: experiences at King Edward VIII Hospital, Durban, South Africa and a review of the literature. *Trop Doct*, Vol.25, No.3 (Jul 1995), pp. 118-123, ISSN 0049-4755

Diao, M., Diop, I.B., Kane, A., Camara, S., Sarr, M., Ba, S.A. & Diouf, S.M. (2004). Electrocardiographic recording of long duration (Holter) of 24 hours during idiopathic cardiomyopathy of the peripartum. *Arch Mal Coeur Vaiss*, Vol.97, No.1 (Jan 2004), pp. 25–30, ISSN 0003-9683

Dickstein, K., Cohen-Solal, A., Filippatos, G., McMurray, J.J.V., Ponikowski, P., Poole-Wilson P.A., Strömberg A., van Veldhuisen D.J., Atar D., Hoes A.W., Keren A., Mebazaa A., Nieminen M., Silvia Giuliana Priori S.G. & Swedberg K. (2008). ESC guidelines for the diagnosis and treatment of acute and chronic heart failure 2008: the Task Force for the diagnosis and treatment of acute and chronic heart failure 2008 of the ESC. *Eur J Heart Fail*, Vol.10, No.10 (Oct 2008), pp. 933-989, ISSN 1388-9842

Dorbala, S., Brozena, S., Logsetty, G., Galatro, K., Homel, P., Ren, JF. & Chaudhry, FA. (2005). Risk stratification of women with peripartum cardiomyopathy at initial presentation: a dobutamine stress echocardiography study. *J Am Soc Echocardiogr*, Vol.18, No.1 (Jan 2005), pp. 45–48, ISSN 0003-2999

Duran, N., Gunes, H., Duran, I., Biteker, M. & Ozkan, M. (2008). Predictors of prognosis in patients with peripartum cardiomyopathy. *Int J Gynaecol Obstet*, Vol.101, No.2 (May 2008), pp. 137–140, ISSN 0020-7292

Egan, R.J., Bisanzom M.C. & Hutson, H.R. (2009). Emergency department evaluation and management of peripartum cardiomyopathy. *J Emerg Med*, Vol.36, No.2 (Feb 2009), pp. 141-147, ISSN 0736-4679

Elkayam, U., Tummala, P.P., Rao, K., Akhter, M.W., Karaalp, I.S., Wani, O.M., Hameed, A., Gviazda, I. & Shotan A. (2001). Maternal and fetal outcomes of subsequent pregnancies in women with peripartum cardiomyopathy. *N Engl J Med*, Vol.344, No.21 (May 2001), pp. 1567–1571, ISSN 0028-4793

Elkayam, U., Akhter, M.W., Singh, H., Khan, S., Bitar, F., Hameed, A. & Shotan, A. (2005). Pregnancy-associated cardiomyopathy: clinical characteristics and a comparison between early and late presentation. *Circulation*, Vol.111, No.6 (Apr 2005), pp. 2050-2055, ISSN 0025-619

Elkayam, U. & Goland, S. (2010). Bromocriptine for the treatment of peripartum cardiomyopathy. *Circulation*, Vol.121, No.13 (Apr 2010), pp. 1463–1464, ISSN 0025-619

Fadouach, S., Matar, N., Meziane, M., Tahiri, A. & Chraibi, N. (1994). Syndrome de Meadows : cardiomyopathie du pèripartum. *Rev Fr Gynecol Obstet*, Vol.89, No.6 (Jun 1994), pp. 335–336, ISSN 1941-2797

Farber, P.A. & Glasgow, L.A. (1970). Viral myocarditis during pregnancy: encephalo-myocarditis virus infection in mice. *Am Heart J*, Vol.80, No.1 (Jul 1970), pp. 96-102, ISSN 0002-870

Ferrero, S., Colombo, B.M., Fenini, F., Abbamonte, L.H. & Arena, E. (2003) Peripartum cardiomyopathy. A review. *Minerva Ginecol*, Vol.55, No.2 (Apr 2003), pp. 151–158, ISSN 0026-4784

Fett, J.D., Carraway, R.D., Dowell, D.L., King, M.E. & Pierre, R. (2002). Peripartum cardiomyopathy in the Hospital Albert Schweitzer District of Haiti. *Am J Obstet Gynecol*, Vol.186, No.5 (May 2002), pp. 1005-1010, ISSN 0002-9378

Fett, J.D., Christie, L.G., Carraway, R.D. & Murphy, J.G. (2005a). Five-year prospective study of the incidence and prognosis of peripartum cardiomyopathy at a single institution. *Mayo Clin Proc*, Vol.80, No.12 (Dec 2005), pp. 1602-1606, ISSN 0025-6196

Fett, J.D., Christie, L.G., Carraway, R.D., Ansari, A.A., Sundstrom, J.B. & Murphy, J.G. (2005b). Unrecognized peripartum cardiomyopathy in Haitian women. *Int J Gynaecol Obstet*, Vol.90, No.2 (Aug 2005), pp. 161–166, ISSN 0020-7292

Fett, J.D. (2006a). Inflammation and virus in dilated cardiomyopathy as indicated by endomyocardial biopsy. *Int J Cardiol*, Vol.112, No.1 (Sep 2006), pp. 125-126, ISSN 0167-5273

Fett JD, Christie LG, Murphy JG. (2006b). Brief communication: Outcomes of subsequent pregnancy after peripartum cardiomyopathy: a case series from Haiti. *Ann Intern Med*, Vol.145, No.1 (Jul 2006), pp. 30–34, ISSN 0003-4819

Fett, J.D. (2008). "Understanding peripartum cardiomyopathy, 2008". *Int. J. Cardiol*, Vol.130, No.1 (Oct 2008), pp. 1–2, ISSN 0167-5273

Fett, J.D. (2009). The role of MRI in peripartum cardiomyopathy. *Int J Cardiol*, Vol.137, No.2 (Oct 2009), pp. 185-186, ISSN 0167-5273

Fett, J.D. (2010). What's next in peripartum cardiomyopathy investigation? *Expert Rev Cardiovasc Ther*, Vol.8, No.6 (Jun 2010), pp. 743-746, ISSN 1477-9072

Fett, J.D. (March 2011). "Validation of a self-test for early diagnosis of heart failure in peripartum cardiomyopathy". *Crit Paths Cardiol*, Vol.10, No.1 (Mar 2011), pp. 44–45, ISSN 1535-282X

Fisher, S.D., Etherington, A., Schwartz, D.B. & Pearson, G.D. (2008). Peripartum cardiomyopathy: An update. *Progr Ped Cardiol*, Vol.25, No.1 (Apr 2008), pp. 79-84, ISSN 1058-9813

Forssell, G., Laska, J., Olofsson, C. Olsson, M. & Mogensen, L. (1994). Peripartum cardiomyopathy: three cases. *J Intern Med*, Vol.235, No.4 (May 1994), pp. 493-496, ISSN 0954-6820

Freedman, N.J. & Lefkowitz, R.J. (2004). Anti-b1-adrenergic receptor antibodies and heart failure: causation, not just correlation. *J Clin Invest*, Vol.113, No.10 (May 2004), pp. 1379-1382, ISSN 0021-9738

Fussell, K.M., Awad, J.A. & Ware, L.B. (2005). "Case of fulminant hepatic failure due to unrecognized peripartum cardiomyopathy". *Crit. Care Med*, Vol.33, No.4 (Apr 2005), pp. 891–893, ISSN 1529-7535

Garrison, E., Hibbard, J.U., Studee, L., Fontana, D., Klibatrick, S. & Briller, J. (2005). Brain natriuretic peptide as a marker for heart disease in pregnancy. *Am J Obstet Gynecol*, Vol.193, No.6 Suppl (Dec 2005), pp. S83, ISSN 0002-9378

Gentry, M.B., Dias, J.K., Luis, A., .Patel, R., Thornton J. & Reed, G.L. (2010). African-American women have a higher risk for developing peripartum cardiomyopathy. *J Am Coll Cardiol*, Vol.55, No.7 (Feb 2010), pp. 654-659, ISSN 0301-4711

Ghuman, N., Rheiner, J., Tendler, B.E. & White, W.B. (2009). Hypertension in the postpartum woman: clinical update for the hypertension specialist. *J Clin Hypertens (Greenwich)*, Vol.11, No.12 (Dec 2009), pp. 726–733, ISSN 1524-6175

Glück, B., Schmidtke, M., Merkle, I., Stelzner, A. & Gemsa, D. (2001). Persistent expression of cytokines in the chronic stage of CVB3-induced myocarditis in NMRI mice. *J Mol Cell Cardiol*, Vol.33, No.9 (Sep 2001), pp. 1615-1626, ISSN 0022-2828

Godsel, L.M., Leon, J.S. & Engman, D.M. (2003). Angiotensin converting enzyme inhibitors and angiotensin II receptor antagonists in experimental myocarditis. *Curr Pharm Des*, Vol.9, No.9 (2003), pp. 723–735, ISSN 1381-6128

Goland, S., Modi, K., Bitar, F., Janmohamed, M., Mirocha, J.M., Czer, L.S., Illum, S., Hatamizadeh, P. & Elkayam, U. (2009). Clinical profile and predictors of complications in peripartum cardiomyopathy. *J Card Fail*, Vol.15, No.8 (Oct 2009), pp. 645–650, ISSN 0091-2700

Gouley, B.A., McMillan, T.M. & Bellet, S. (1937). Idiopathic myocardial degeneration associated with pregnancy and especially the puerperium. *Am J Med Sci*, Vol.194 (1937), pp. 185-189, ISSN 0002-9629

Habedank, D., Kuhnle, Y., Elgeti, T., Dudenhausen, J.W., Haverkamp, W. & Dietz, R. (2008). Recovery from peripartum cardiomyopathy after treatment with bromocriptine. *Eur J Heart Fail*, Vol.10, No.11 (Nov 2008), pp. 1149-1151, ISSN 1388-9842

Habli, M., O'Brien, T., Nowack, E., Khoury, S., Barton, J.R. & Sibai, B. (2008). Peripartum cardiomyopathy: prognostic factors for long-term maternal outcome. *Am J Obstet Gynecol*, Vol.199, No.4 (Oct 2008), pp. 415.e1–5, ISSN 0025-6196

Hameed, A.B., Chan, K., Ghamsary, M. & Elkayam, U. (2009). Longitudinal changes in the B-type natriuretic peptide levels in normal pregnancy and post partum. *Clin Cardiol*, Vol.32, No.8 (Aug 2009), pp. E60–E62, ISSN 0160-9289

Helms, A.K., & Kittner, S.J. (2005). Pregnancy and stroke. *CNS Spectr*, Vol.10, No.7 (Jul 2005), pp. 580–587, ISSN 1092-8529

Hershberger, R.E., Lindenfeld, J., Mestroni, L., Seidman, C.E., Taylor, M.R. & Towbin, J.A. (2009). Genetic evaluation of cardiomyopathy: a Heart Failure Society of America practice guideline. *J Card Fail*, Vol. 15, No.2 (Mar 2009), pp. 83-97, ISSN 0091-2700

Hibbard, J.U., Lindheimer, M., Lang, R.M. (1999). A modified definition for peripartum cardiomyopathy and prognosis based on echocardiography. *Obstet Gynecol*, Vol.94, No.2 (Aug 1999), pp. 311–316, ISSN 0029-7844

Hilfiker-Kleiner, D., Kaminski, K., Podewski, E., Bonda, T., Schaefer, A., Sliwa, K., Forster, O., Quint, A., Landmesser, U., Doerries, C., Luchtefeld, M., Poli, V., Schneider, M.D., Balligand, J.L., Desjardins, F., Ansari, A., Struman, I., Nguyen, N.Q., Zschemisch, N.H., Klein, G., Heusch, G., Schulz, R., Hilfiker, A. & Drexler, H. (2007a). A cathepsin D-cleaved 16 kDa form of prolactin mediates postpartum cardiomyopathy. *Cell*, Vol.128, No.3, (Feb 2007), pp. 589-600, ISSN 0092-8674

Hilfiker-Kleiner, D., Meyer, G.P., Schieffer, E., Goldmann, B., Podewski, E., Struman, I., Fischer, P. & Drexler, H. (2007b). Recovery from postpartum cardiomyopathy in 2 patients by blocking prolactin release with bromocriptine. *J Am Coll Cardiol*, Vol.50, No.24 (Dec 2007), pp. 2354-2355, ISSN 0735-1097

Hilfiker-Kleiner, D., Sliwa, K. & Drexler, H. (2008). Peripartum Cardiomyopathy: Recent Insights in its Pathophysiology. *Trends Cardiovasc Med*, Vol.18, No.5 (July 2008), pp. 173–179, ISSN 1050-1738

Hopp, L., Haider, B. & Iffy, L. (1996). Myocardial infarction postpartum in patients taking bromocriptine for the prevention of breast engorgement. *Int J Cardiol*, Vol.57, No.3 (Dec 1996), pp. 227–232, ISSN 0167-5273

Horwitz, M.S., Knudsen, M., Fine, C., Fine, C. & Sarvetnick, N. (2007). Transforming growth factor-beta inhibits cocksackievirus mediated autoimmune myocarditis. *Viral Immunol*, Vol.19, No.4 (Jan 2007), pp. 722–733, ISSN 0882-8245

Hu, C.L., Li, Y.B., Zou, Y.G., Zhang, J.M., Chen, J.B., Liu, J., Tang, Y.H., Tang, Q.Z. & Huang, C.X. (2007). Troponin T measurement can predict persistent left ventricular dysfunction in peripartum cardiomyopathy. *Heart*, Vol.93, No.4 (Apr 2007), pp. 488–490, ISSN 1355-6037

Hunt, S.A., Abraham, W.T., Chin, M.H., Feldman, A.M., Francis, G.S., Ganiats, T.G., Jessup, M., Konstam, M.A., Mancini, D.M., Michl, K., Oates, J.A., Rahko, P.S., Silver, M.A., Stevenson, L.W. & Yancy, C.W. (2009). 2009 Focused update incorporated into the ACC/AHA 2005 guidelines for the diagnosis and management of heart failure in adults: a report of the American College of Cardiology Foundation/ American Heart Association Task Force on Practice Guidelines. *Circulation*, Vol.119, No.14 (Apr 2009), pp. e391–479, ISSN 0006-3363

Jahns, R., Boivin, V., Hein, L., . Triebel, S., Angermann, C.E., Ertl, G. & Lohse, M.J. (2004). Direct evidence for a b1-adrenergic receptor directed autoimmune attack as a cause of idiopathic dilated cardiomyopathy. *J Clin Invest*, Vol.113, No.10 (May 2004), pp. 1419-1429, ISSN 0021-9738

Jahns, B.G., Stein, W., Hilfiker-Kleiner, D., Pieske, B. & Emons, G. (2008). Peripartum cardiomyopathy–a new treatment option by inhibition of prolactin secretion. *Am J Obstet Gynecol*, Vol.199, No.4 (Oct 2008), pp. e5–e6, ISSN 0002-9378

Jha, P., Jha, S. & Millane, T.A. (2005). Peripartum cardiomyopathy complicated by pulmonary embolism and pulmonary hypertension. *Eur J Obstet Gynecol Reprod Biol*, Vol.123, No.1 (Nov 2005), pp. 121–123, ISSN 0301-2115

Kane, A., Dia, A.A., Diouf, A., Dia, D., Diop, I.B., Moreau, J.C., Faye, E.O., Sarr, M., Ba, S.A., Diadhiou, F. & Diouf, S.M. (2001). La myocardiopathie idiopathique du péripartum: étude prospective échocardiographique. *Ann Cardiol Angeiol*, Vol.50, No.6 (Oct 2001), pp. 305–311, ISSN 0003-3928

Kawano, H., Tsuneto, A., Koide, Y., Tasaki, H,. Sueyoshi, E., Sakamoto, I. & Hayashi, T. (2008). Magnetic resonance imaging in a patient with peripartum cardiomyopathy. *Intern Med*, Vol.47, No.2 (Jan 2008), pp. 97–102, ISSN 1444-0903

Kim, Y.J., Park, H.S., Park, M.H., Suh, S.H. & Pang, M.G. (2005). Oxidative stress-related gene polymorphism and the risk of preeclampsia. *Eur J Obst. Gyn. Reprod. Biol.*, Vol.119, No.1 (Mar 2005), pp. 42–46, ISSN 1360-9947

Kothari, S.S. (1997). Aetiopathogenesis of peripartum cardiomyopathy: prolactin–selenium interaction? *Int J Cardiol*, Vol.60, No.1 (June 1997), pp. 111–114, ISSN 0167-5273

Kühl, U., Pauschinger, M., Noutsias, M., Seeberg, B., Bock, T., Lassner, D., Poller, W., Kandolf, R. & Schultheiss, H.P. (2005a). High prevalence of viral genomes and multiple viral infections in the myocardium of adults with "idiopathic" left ventricular dysfunction. *Circulation*, Vol.111, No.7 (Feb 2005), pp. 887-893, ISSN 0009-7322

Kühl, U., Pauschinger, M., Seeberg, B., Lassner, D., Noutsias, M., Poller, W. & Schultheiss, H.P. (2005b). Viral persistence in the myocardium is associated with progressive cardiac dysfunction. *Circulation*, Vol.112, No.13 (Sep 2005), pp. 1965–1970, ISSN 0009-7322

Lampert, M.B. & Lang, R.M. (1995). Peripartum cardiomyopathy. *Am Heart J*, Vol.130, No.4 (Oct 1995), pp. 860–870, ISSN 0002-8703

Lampert, M.B., Weinert, L., Hibbard, J., Korcarz, C., Lindheimer, M. & Lang, R.M. (1997). Contractile reserve in patients with peripartum cardiomyopathy and recovered left ventricular function. *Am J Obstet Gynecol*, Vol.176, No.1 (Jan 1997), pp. 189-195, ISSN 0002-9378

Lang, C., Sauter, M., Szalay, G., Racchi, G., Grassi, G., Rainaldi, G., Mercatanti, A., Lang, F., Kandolf, R. & Klingel, K. (2008). Connective tissue growth factor: a crucial cytokine-mediating cardiac fibrosis in ongoing enterovirus myocarditis. *J Mol Med*, Vol.86, No.1 (Jan 2008), pp. 49-60, ISSN 0946-2716

Lasinska-Kowara, M., Dudziak, M. & Suchorzewska, J. (2001). "Two cases of postpartum cardiomyopathy initially misdiagnosed for pulmonary embolism". *Can J Anaesth*, Vol.48, No.8 (Sep 2001), pp. 773–777, ISSN 0832-610X

Leurent, G., Baruteau, A.E., Larralde, A., Ollivier, R., Schleich, J.M., Boulmier, D., Bedossa, M., Langella, B. & Le Breton, H. (2009). Contribution of cardiac MRI in the comprehension of peripartum cardiomyopathy pathogenesis. *Int J Cardiol*, Vol.132, No.3 (Mar 2009), pp. e91–93, ISSN 0301-471

Lindheimer, M.D. & Katz, A.I. (1973). Sodium and diuretics in pregnancy. *N Engl J Med*, Vol.288, No.17 (Apr 1973), pp. 891–894, ISSN 0028-4793

Maron, B.J., Towbin, J.A., Thiene, G., Antzelevitch, C., Corrado, D., Arnett, D., Moss, A.J., Seidman, C.E. & Young, J.B. (2006). Contemporary definitions and classification of the cardiomyopathies: an American Heart Association Scientific Statement from the Council on Clinical Cardiology, Heart Failure and Transplantation Committee; Quality of Care and Outcomes Research and Functional Genomics and Translational Biology Interdisciplinary Working Groups; and Council on Epidemiology and Prevention. *Circulation*, Vol.113, No.14 (Apr 2006), pp. 1807-1816, ISSN 0009-7322

Meyer, G.P., Labidi, S., Podewski, E., Sliwa, K., Drexler, H. & Hilfiker-Kleiner, D. (2010). Bromocriptine treatment associated with recovery from peripartum cardiomyopathy in siblings: two case reports. *J Med Case Rep*, Vol.4, No.4 (Mar 2010), pp. 80, ISSN 1752-1947

Midei, M., DeMent, S., Feldman, A., Hutchins, G.M. & Baughman, K.L. (1990). Peripartum myocarditis and cardiomyopathy. *Circulation*, Vol. 81, No. 3 (Mar 1990), pp. 922-928, ISSN 0009-7322

Mielniczuk, L.M., Williams, K., Davis, D.R., Tang, A.S., Lemery, R., Green, M.S., Gollob, M.H., Haddad, H. & Birnie, D.H. (2006). Frequency of peripartum cardiomyopathy. *Am J Cardiol*, Vol.97, No.12 (Jun 2006), pp. 1765-1768, ISSN 0002-9149

Modi, K.A., Illum, S., Jariatul, K., Caldito, G. & Reddy, P.C. (2009). Poor outcome of indigent patients with peripartum cardiomyopathy in the United States. *Am J Obstet Gynecol*, Vol.201, No.2 (Aug 2009), pp. 171.e1–5, ISSN 0002-9378

Moioli, M., Menada, M.V., Bentivoglio, G. & Ferrero, S. (2010). Peripartum cardiomyopathy. *Arch Gynecol Obstet*, Vol. 281, No. 2 (Feb 2010), pp. 183-188, ISSN 0932-0067

Morales, A., Painter, T, Li, R., Siegfried, J.D., Li, D., Norton, N. & Hershberger, R.E. (2010). Rare variant mutations in pregnancy-associated or peripartum cardiomyopathy. *Circulation*, Vol.121, No.20 (May 2010), pp. 2176–2182, ISSN 0009-7322

Mouquet, F., Lions, C., de Groote, P., Bouabdallaoui, N., Willoteaux, S., Dagorn, J., Deruelle, P., Lamblin, N., Bauters, C. & Beregi, J.P. (2008). Characterisation of peripartum cardiomyopathy by cardiac magnetic resonance imaging. *Eur Radiol*, Vol.18, No.12 (Dec 2008), pp.:2765–2769, ISSN 0033-8419

Muldowney, J.A. III., Schoenhard, J.A. & Benge, C.D. (2009). The clinical pharmacology of eplerenone. *Expert Opin Drug Metab Toxicol*, Vol.5, No.4 (Apr 2009), pp. 425-432, ISSN 1742-5255

Murali, S. & Baldisseri, M.R. (2005). Peripartum cardiomyopathy. *Crit Care Med*, Vol.33, No.10 (Suppl) (Oct 2005), pp. S340-S346, ISSN 0090-3493

Nagafuchi, H., Suzuki, N., Kaneko, A., Asai, T. & Sakane, T. (1999). Prolactin locally produced by synovium infiltrating T lymphocytes induces excessive synovial cell functions in patients with rheumatoid arthritis. *J Rheumatol*, Vol.26, No.9 (Sep 1999), pp. 1890–1900, ISSN 0315-162x

Narula, J., Kolodgie, F.D. & Virmani, R. (2000). Apoptosis and cardiomyopathy. *Curr Opin Cardiol*, Vol.15, No.3 (May 2000), pp. 183-188, ISSN 0268-4705

Negoro, S., Kunisada, K., Fujio, Y., Funamoto, M., Darville, M.I., Eizirik, D.L., Osugi, T., Izumi, M., Oshima, Y., Nakaoka, Y., Hirota, H., Kishimoto, T. & Yamauchi-Takihara, K. (2001). Activation of signal transducer and activator of transcription 3 protects cardiomyocytes from hypoxia/reoxygenation-induced oxidative stress through the upregulation of manganese superoxide dismutase. *Circulation*, Vol.104, No.9 (Aug 2001), pp. 979-981, ISSN 1524-4539

Nkoua, J.L., Kimbaly-Kaky, G., Onkani, A.H., Kandosi, S. & Bouramoue, C. (1991). La myocardiopathie du post-partum. À propos de 24 cas. *Cardiol Trop*, Vol. 17, No. 67 (1991), pp. 105-110, ISSN 1995-1892

Ntusi, N.B.A. & Mayosi, B.M. Aetiology and risk factors of peripartum cardiomyopathy: A systematic review. *Int J Cardiology*, Vol.131, No.2 (Jan 2009), pp. 168-179, ISSN 0167-5273

Oakley, C., Child, A., Iung, B., Presbitero, P., Tornos, P., Klein, W., Garcia, M.A.A., Blomstrom-Lundqvist, C., de Backer, G., Dargie, H., Deckers, J., Flather, M., Hradec, J., Mazzotta, G., Oto, A., Parkhomenko, A., Silber, S., Torbicki, A., Trappe, H.J., Dean, V., & Poumeyrol-Jumeau, D. (2003). Expert consensus document on management of cardiovascular diseases during pregnancy.Task force on the management of cardiovascular diseases during pregnancy of the European society of cardiology. *Eur Heart J*, Vol.24, No.8 (Apr 2003), pp. 761-781, ISSN 0195-668x

Pauschinger, M., Rutschow, W., Chandrasekharan, K., Westermann, D., Weitz, A., Peter, S.L,, Zeichhardt, H., Poller, W., Noutsias, M., Li, J., Schultheiss, H.P. & Tschope, C. (2005). Carvedilol improves left ventricular function in murine coxsackievirus-induced active myocarditis associated with reduced myocardial interleukin-1beta and MMP-8 expression and a modulated immune response. *Eur J Heart Fail*, Vol.7, No.4 (Jun 2005), pp. 444–452, ISSN 1388-9842

Pearson, G.D., Veille, J.C., Rahimtoola, S., Hsia, J., Oakley, C.M., Hosenpud, J.D., Ansari, A. & Baughman, K.L. (2000). Peripartum cardiomyopathy. National Heart Lung and Blood Institute and Office of Rare Diseases (National Institutes of Health)

workshop recommendations and review. *JAMA*, Vol.283, No.9 (Mar 2000), pp. 1183-1888, ISSN 0098-7484

Pierce, J.A., Price, B.O. & Joyce, J.W. (1963). Familial occurrence of postpartal heart failure. *Arch Intern Med*, Vol.111, No.5 (May 1963), pp. 151-155, ISSN 0003-9926

Porak C. (1880). De l'influence reciproque de la grossesse et des maladies du Couer, thesis, Paris, 1880

Potapov, E.V., Loforte, A., Weng, Y., Jurmann, M., Pasic, M., Drews, T., Loebe, M., Hennig, E., Krabatsch, T., Koster, A., Lehmkuhl, H.B. &, Hetzer, R. (2008). Experience with over 1000 implanted ventricular assist devices. *J Card Surg*, Vol.23, No.3 (May-Jun 2008), pp. 185–194, ISSN 0886-0440

Pyatt, R.J. & Dubey, G. (2011). Peripartum cardiomyopathy: current understanding, comprehensive management review and new developments. *Postgrad Med J*, Vol.87, No.1023 (Jan 2011), pp. 34-39, ISSN 1560-5876

Ramaraj, R. & Sorrell, V.L. (2009). Peripartum cardiomyopathy: causes, diagnosis, and treatment. *Clev Clin J Med*, Vol.76, No.5 (May 2009), pp. 289-296, ISSN 0891-1150

Rasmusson, K.D., Stehlik, J., Brown, R.N., Renlund, D.G., Wagoner, L.E., Torre-Amione, G., Folsom, J.W., Silber, D.H. & Kirklin, J.K. (2007). Longterm outcomes of cardiac transplantation for peri-partum cardiomyopathy: a multiinstitutional analysis. *J Heart Lung Transplant*, Vol.26, No.11 (Nov 2007), pp. 1097–1104, ISSN 1053-2498

Ritchie, C. (1849). Clinical contribution to the pathology, diagnosis and treatment of certain chronic diseases in the heart. *Edinburgh Med Surg*, Vol.2, pp. 333, ISSN 0003-2999

Rizeq, M.N., Rickenbache, P.R., Fowler, M.B. & Billingham ,M.E. (1994). Incidence of myocarditis in peripartum cardiomyopathy. *Am J Cardiol*, Vol.74, No.5 (Sep 1994), pp. 474-477, ISSN 0002-9149

Roberg, K. & Ollinger, K. (1998). Oxidative stress causes relocation of the lysosomal enzyme cathepsin D with ensuing apoptosis in neonatal rat cardiomyocytes. *Am J Pathol*, Vol.152, No.1 (May 1998), pp. 1151-1156, ISSN 0002-9440

Robson, S.C., Hunter, S., Boys, R.J. & Dunlop, W. (1989). Serial study of factors influencing changes in cardiac output during human pregnancy. *Am J Physiol Heart Circ Physiol*, Vol.256, No.4 (Apr 1989), pp. 1060-1065, ISSN 0363-6135

Sliwa, K., Skudicky, D., Bergemann, A., Cand,y G., Puren, A. & Sareli, P. (2000). Peripartum cardiomyopathy: analysis of clinical outcome, left ventricular function, plasma levels of cytokines and Fas/APO-1. *J Am Coll Cardiol*, Vol.35, No.3 (Mar 2000), pp. 701–705, ISSN :0735-1097

Sliwa, K., Skukicky, D., Candy, G., Bergemann, A., Hopley, M. & Sareli, P. (2002). The addition of pentoxifylline to conventional therapy improves outcome in patients with peripartum cardiomyopathy. *Eur J Heart Fail*, Vol.4, No.3 (Jun 2002), pp. 305–309, ISSN 1388-9842

Sliwa, K., Fett, J. & Elkayam, U. (2006a). Peripartum cardiomyopathy. *Lancet*, Vol.368, No.9536 (Aug 2006), pp. 687-693, ISSN 0140-6736

Sliwa, K., Forster, O., Libhaber, E., Fett, J.D., Sundstrom, J.B., Hilfiker-Kleiner, D. & Ansari, A.A. (2006b). Peripartum cardiomyopathy: inflammatory markers as predictors of outcome in 100 prospectively studied patients. *Eur Heart J*, Vol.27, No.4 (Feb 2006), pp. 441–446, ISSN 0195-668X

Sliwa, K., Hilfiker-Kleiner, D., Petrie, M.C., Mebazaa, A., Pieske, B., Buchmann, E., Regitz-Zagrosek, V., Schaufelberger, M., Tavazzi, L,, van Veldhuisen, D.J., Watkins, H.,

Shah, A.J., Seferovic, P.M., Elkayam, U., Pankuweit, S., Papp, Z., Mouquet, F. & McMurray, J.J. (2010a). Current state of knowledge on aetiology, diagnosis, management, and therapy of peripartum cardiomyopathy: a position statement from the Heart Failure Association of the European Society of Cardiology Working Group on peripartum cardiomyopathy. *Eur J Heart Fail*, Vol.12, No.8 (Aug 2010), pp. 767-778, ISSN 1388-9842

Sliwa, K., Blauwet, L., Tibazarwa, K. Libhaber, E., Smedema, J.P., Becker, A., McMurray, J., Yamac, H., Labidi, S., Struman, I. & Hilfiker-Kleiner, D. (2010b). Evaluation of bromocriptine in the treatment of acute severe peripartum cardiomyopathy. A proof-of-concept pilot study. *Circulation*, Vol.121, No.13 (Mar 2010), pp. 1465-1473, ISSN 1524-4539

Srichai, M.B., Junor, C., Rodriguez, L.L., Stillman, A.E., Grimm, R.A., Lieber, M.L., Weaver, J.A., Smedira, N.G. & White, R.D. (2006). Clinical, imaging, and pathological characteristics of left ventricular thrombus: a comparison of contrast-enhanced magnetic resonance imaging, transthoracic echocardiography, and transesophageal echocardiography with surgical or pathological validation. *Am Heart J*, Vol.152, No.1 (Jul 2006), pp. 75–84, ISSN 0002-8703

Thorne, S., MacGregor, A. & Nelson-Piercy, C. (2006). Risks of contraception and pregnancy in heart disease. *Heart*, Vol.92, No.10 (Oct 2006), pp. 1520–1525, ISSN 1355-6037

Toescu, V., Nuttall, S.L., Martin, U., Kendall, M.J. & Dunne, F. (2002). Oxidative stress and normal pregnancy. *Clin Endocrinol (Oxf)*, Vol. 57, No. 5 (Nov 2002), pp. 609-613, ISSN 0300-0664

Torbicki, A., Perrier, A., Konstandinides, S., Galiè, N., Pruszczyk, P., Bengel, F., Brady, A.J, Ferreira, D., Janssens, U., Klepetko, W., Mayer, E., Remy-Jardin, M. & Bassand, J.P. (2008). Guidelines on the diagnosis and management of acute pulmonary embolism. The Task Force for the Diagnosis and Management of Acute Pulmonary Embolism of the European Society of Cardiology. *Eur Heart J*, Vol.29, No.18 (Sep 2008), pp. 2276-2315, ISSN 0195-668x

van Spaendonck-Zwarts, K., van Tintelen, J., van Veldhuisen, D.J., van der Werf, R., Jongbloed, J.D., Paulus, W.J., Dooijes, D. & van den Berg, M.P. (2010). Peripartum cardiomyopathy as part of familial dilated cardiomyopathy. *Circulation*, Vol.121, No.20 (May 2010), pp. 2169–2175, ISSN 0009-7322

Walsh, J.J., Burch, C.E., Black, W.C., Ferrans, V.J. & Hibbs, R.G. (1965). Idiopathic myocardiopathy of the peripartum. *Circulation*, Vol.32 (Jul 1965), pp. 19-31, ISSN 0009-7322

Warraich, R.S., Sliwa, K., Damasceno, A., Carraway, R., Sundrom, B., Arif, G., Essop, R., Ansari, A., Fett, J. & Yacoub, M. (2005). Impact of pregnancy-related heart failure on humoral immunity: clinical relevance of G3-subclass immunoglobulins in peripartum cardiomyopathy. *Am Heart J*, Vol.150, No.2 (Aug 2005), pp. 263-269, ISSN 0002-870

Webb, J.A., Thomsen, H.S. & Morcos, S.K. (2005). The use of iodinated and gadolinium contrast media during pregnancy and lactation. *Eur Radiol*, Vol.15, No.6 (Jun 2005), pp. 1234–1240, ISSN 0033-8419

Weinblatt, M., Singer, M.A. & Iqbal, I. (1995). Peripartum cardiomyopathy: a case report and review of literature. *Primary Care Update for Ob Gyns*, Vol.2, No.2 (Mar-Apr 1995), pp 59–62, ISSN 1068-607X V

Wencker, D., Chandra, M., Nguyen, K., Miao, W., Garantziotis, S., Factor, S.M., Shirani, J., Armstrong, R.C. & Kitsis, R.N. (2003). A mechanistic role for cardiac myocyte apoptosis in heart failure. *J Clin Invest*, Vol.111, No.10 (May 2003), pp. 1497-1504, ISSN 0895-4356

Whitehead, S.J., Berg, C.J. & Chang J. (2003). Pregnancy related mortality due to cardiomyopathy: United States, 1991-1997. *Obstet Gynecol*, Vol.102, No.6 (Dec 2003), pp. 1326-1331, ISSN 0029-7844

Wittstein, I.S., Thiemann, D.R., Lima, J.A.C., Baughman, K.L., Schulman, S.P., Gerstenblith, G., Wu, K.C., Rade, J.J., Bivalacqua, T.J. & Champion, H.C. (2005). Neurohumoral features of myocardial stunning due to sudden emotional stress. *N Engl J Med*, Vol. 352, No.6 (Feb 2005), pp. 539-548, ISSN 0028-4793

Yahagi, N., Kumon, K. & Nakatani, T. (1994). Peripartum cardiomyopathy and tachycardia followed by multiple organ failure. *Anesth Analg*, Vol.79, No.3 (Sep 1994), pp. 581-582, ISSN 0003-2999

Yang, H.S., Hong, Y.S., Rim, S.J. & Yu, S.H. (2007). Extracorporeal membrane oxygenation in a patient with peripartum cardiomyopathy. *Ann Thorac Surg*, Vol.84, No.1 (Jul 2007), pp. 262-264, ISSN 0003-4975

Zimmermann, O., Kochs, M., Zwaka, T.P., Kaya, Z., Lepper, P.M., Bienek-Ziolkowski, M., Hoher, M., Hombach, V. & Torzewski, J. (2005). Myocardial biopsy based classification and treatment in patients with dilated cardiomyopathy. *Int J Cardiol*, Vol.104, No.1 (Sep 2005), pp. 92-100, ISSN 0167-5273

Zimmerman, H., Bose, R., Smith, R. & Copeland, J.G. Treatment of Peripartum Cardiomyopathy With Mechanical Assist Devices and Cardiac Transplantation. *Ann Thorac Surg*, Vol. 89, No.4 (Apr 2010), pp. 1211-1217, ISSN 0003-4975.

Permissions

The contributors of this book come from diverse backgrounds, making this book a truly international effort. This book will bring forth new frontiers with its revolutionizing research information and detailed analysis of the nascent developments around the world.

We would like to thank Josef Veselka, MD, PhD, for lending his expertise to make the book truly unique. He has played a crucial role in the development of this book. Without his invaluable contribution this book wouldn't have been possible. He has made vital efforts to compile up to date information on the varied aspects of this subject to make this book a valuable addition to the collection of many professionals and students.

This book was conceptualized with the vision of imparting up-to-date information and advanced data in this field. To ensure the same, a matchless editorial board was set up. Every individual on the board went through rigorous rounds of assessment to prove their worth. After which they invested a large part of their time researching and compiling the most relevant data for our readers. Conferences and sessions were held from time to time between the editorial board and the contributing authors to present the data in the most comprehensible form. The editorial team has worked tirelessly to provide valuable and valid information to help people across the globe.

Every chapter published in this book has been scrutinized by our experts. Their significance has been extensively debated. The topics covered herein carry significant findings which will fuel the growth of the discipline. They may even be implemented as practical applications or may be referred to as a beginning point for another development. Chapters in this book were first published by InTech; hereby published with permission under the Creative Commons Attribution License or equivalent.

The editorial board has been involved in producing this book since its inception. They have spent rigorous hours researching and exploring the diverse topics which have resulted in the successful publishing of this book. They have passed on their knowledge of decades through this book. To expedite this challenging task, the publisher supported the team at every step. A small team of assistant editors was also appointed to further simplify the editing procedure and attain best results for the readers.

Our editorial team has been hand-picked from every corner of the world. Their multi-ethnicity adds dynamic inputs to the discussions which result in innovative outcomes. These outcomes are then further discussed with the researchers and contributors who give their valuable feedback and opinion regarding the same. The feedback is then collaborated with the researches and they are edited in a comprehensive manner to aid the understanding of the subject.

Apart from the editorial board, the designing team has also invested a significant amount of their time in understanding the subject and creating the most relevant covers. They scrutinized every image to scout for the most suitable representation of the subject and create an appropriate cover for the book.

The publishing team has been involved in this book since its early stages. They were actively engaged in every process, be it collecting the data, connecting with the contributors or procuring relevant information. The team has been an ardent support to the editorial, designing and production team. Their endless efforts to recruit the best for this project, has resulted in the accomplishment of this book. They are a veteran in the field of academics and their pool of knowledge is as vast as their experience in printing. Their expertise and guidance has proved useful at every step. Their uncompromising quality standards have made this book an exceptional effort. Their encouragement from time to time has been an inspiration for everyone.

The publisher and the editorial board hope that this book will prove to be a valuable piece of knowledge for researchers, students, practitioners and scholars across the globe.

List of Contributors

Bhulan Kumar Singh, Krishna Kolappa Pillai and Syed Ehtaishamul Haque
Department of Pharmacology, Faculty of Pharmacy, Hamdard University, New Delhi, India

Kanchan Kohli
Department of Pharmaceutics, Faculty of Pharmacy, Hamdard University, New Delhi, India

Mirela Ovreiu and Dan Simon
Cleveland Clinic Foundation, Cleveland State University, United States

M. Obadah Al Chekakie
University of Colorado, Cheyenne Regional Medical Center, United States

Mototsugu Nishii and Tohru Izumi
Kitasato University School of Medicine, Japan

Josef Veselka
Department of Cardiology, 2nd Medical School, Charles University, University Hospital Motol, Prague, Czech Republic

Luis E. Alday and Eduardo Moreyra
Divisions of Cardiology, Hospital Aeronáutico and Sanatorio Allende, Córdoba, Argentina

Elisabete Nave Leal
Polytechnic Institute of Lisbon /School of Health Technology of Lisbon, Portugal

José Luís Pais Ribeiro
University of Porto/Faculty of Psychology and Educational Sciences, Portugal

Mário Martins Oliveira
Lisbon Central Hospital Center, Santa Marta Hospital, Portugal

Viviana Aursulesei and Mihai Dan Datcu
University of Medicine and Pharmacy "Gr. T. Popa", Iasi, Romania

Printed in the USA
CPSIA information can be obtained
at www.ICGtesting.com
JSHW011355221024
72173JS00003B/286